The AIMS Guide to

Resolution After Birth

An AIMS publication

Principal Author: Shane Ridley

AIMS Trustee and Publications Secretary

Published by AIMS

www.aims.org.uk

publications@aims.org.uk

Tel: 0300 365 0663

© AIMS 2020

Association for Improvements in the Maternity Services

Registered Charity number 1157845

ISBN: 978-1-874413448

A catalogue record for this book is available from the British Library.

Printed in the Czech Republic by Printo

About AIMS

The Association for Improvements in the Maternity Services (AIMS) has been at the forefront of the childbirth movement since 1960. It is a volunteer-run charity and most of its work is carried out by volunteers without payment.

AIMS' day-to-day work includes providing independent support and information about maternity choices and raising awareness of current research on childbirth and related issues. AIMS actively supports parents, midwives, doctors and birth workers who recognise that, for the majority of women, birth is a normal rather than a medical event. AIMS campaigns tirelessly on many issues covered by the Human Rights legislation.

AIMS campaigns internationally, nationally and locally for better births for all, protecting human rights in childbirth and the provision of objective, evidence based information to enable informed decision making.

AIMS Mission

"We support all maternity service users to navigate the system as it exists, and campaign for a system which truly meets the needs of all."

AIMS Equality, Diversity and Inclusivity Statement

AIMS Equality, Diversity and Inclusivity Statement is available on the AIMS website at *www.aims.org.uk/general/aims-equality-diversity-and-inclusivity-statement.*

AIMS promotes equality, values diversity and challenges discrimination and with this statement we make a commitment to do so irrespective of characteristics. Freedom of expression is fundamental to AIMS and we will endeavour to publish diverse voices and wide-ranging opinions.

AIMS will work towards ensuring that all our written works will be made available in a variety of formats to meet different needs and that the language is inclusive to all.

AIMS wishes to support everyone throughout their pregnancy, ensuring that they are protected, included, celebrated and retain autonomy over their bodies.

Acknowledgements

Whilst I am the principal author and researcher for Resolution, I have worked closely with colleagues, notably Winsa Dai, AIMS Member and Volunteer, who added her expertise and knowledge throughout the book, Emma Ashworth, AIMS Trustee, who helped considerably with the chapter on Consent and Becky Talbot, AIMS Member, Volunteer and doula, who assisted with the Fear of Referral to Children's Services.

I invited the following people from other charities and networks to author chapters in the book and I am very grateful for their input and support, and thank them warmly. The guest authors are Elizabeth Prochaska, Maria Booker, Dr Rebecca Moore and Clea Harmer.

Elizabeth Prochaska is founder and Chair of Trustees of Birthrights and a barrister specialising in public and human rights law. She was formerly Legal Director of the Equality and Human Rights Commission. She has a particular interest and expertise in women's rights relating to pregnancy and childbirth and regularly advises women and health professionals in this area. She has lectured on childbirth rights around the world, working with lawyers and campaigners to promote women's dignity and autonomy.

Maria Booker is Programmes Director for the human rights in childbirth charity Birthrights and is responsible for the organisation's policy and legal hub, as well as Birthrights' training programme for healthcare professionals and peer supporters. Prior to Birthrights, Maria was the UK Managing Director for Maternity Neighbourhood – a US midwife-led company that had developed a woman-centred, electronic, shared maternity record. She also led the development of the website *Which? Birth Choice* for *Which?* Maria is a member and former Chair of her local Maternity Voices Partnership.

Dr Rebecca Moore is a Consultant Perinatal Psychiatrist and birth trauma expert who hosts an annual birth trauma conference in London each year. Rebecca is co-founder of Make Birth Better, a unique collaboration of parents and professionals dedicated to reducing the life changing impact of birth trauma through education, campaigning and research.

Clea Harmer joined Sands in July 2016 as their Chief Executive. She is passionate about the importance of peer support and in enabling parents to make decisions that are right for them. Her background in Higher Education and Medicine has shaped her belief in the importance of using research to create positive change.

Liz Thomas joined AvMA in 1989 and has been involved in all aspects of AvMA's work. As Policy & Research Manager, Liz is responsible, in conjunction with the Chief Executive, for developing and promoting AvMA's policy work, and has a particular interest in patient safety in obstetrics. Her other key role is overseeing the administration of the AvMA Specialist Clinical Negligence Panel, a highly respected accreditation scheme for specialist lawyers.

Like all AIMS publications, this book has benefitted immensely from the critical comments and suggestions of a group of AIMS Volunteers. It is this approach, drawing on the knowledge and insight of both expert and lay readers, which ensures that AIMS books meet the needs of our main audience, the individual maternity service user, as well as providing valuable information to those who support them.

I am very grateful for the tireless support of our editor, Alison Melvin, who also typeset the manuscript. A big thank you to Chloe Bayfield, former AIMS Trustee, for proofreading. And final thanks to our printer in the Czech Republic, Daniel Zabek, who created the book itself.

My inspiration for the book came from a previous AIMS booklet called Making a Complaint, written and updated on more than one occasion by Beverley Lawrence Beech, former Chair of AIMS. In these times when 'medicalised' birth is increasingly the norm, within a culture of blame, we realised that seeking resolution for a birth which didn't go to plan isn't always about making a complaint; it can take a lot more than that.

I hope this book helps by signposting the different ways of seeking resolution for you or those you are helping. Alternatively, you may want to read this book before or during your pregnancy to increase your awareness of some of the pitfalls of the maternity system!

Shane Ridley
AIMS Trustee, Publications Secretary and Principal Author

Contents

Introduction

Resolution is the noun from the Latin 'resolvere' meaning 'to loosen, undo, explain'. We use it to mean 'the settlement of an issue', 'completion or conclusion of conflicts', 'having a determination', 'expressing an opinion', 'resolving on a course of action'. This book is about helping people to seek resolution for any regret or trauma, emotional or physical, triggered by a birthing experience.

You can read this book as part of preparation for pregnancy, to remind you of your rights and to bring you an awareness of the potential pitfalls of the maternity services. If there are occasions when you feel pressurised into a particular action to do with your care, I hope it will impress upon you that all medical procedures require your consent, and that this is key to being able to control what happens. There is a full chapter on how to give your consent to any procedure offered to you. As well as any physical side-effects of any intervention or medication, we need to understand the psychological and emotional ones too – affecting both ourselves and our babies.

This is also a reference book – to be dipped into when necessary. It contains information about who you can talk to if you have had an upsetting experience, about who to write to, about how to make a formal complaint or to raise a concern, and many other options, with signposts to support services and organisations available to meet various needs.

In some cases, you may have to make a complaint prior to the birth to get the service that you need for you or your baby. If this is your situation, go straight to Chapter 8 and look for information about the Professional Midwifery Advocate who should be able to support you. Or you can use the complaints procedure if you have been denied a service that you have a right to, and you have already spoken to the person or organisation who should provide the service and are not satisfied with their response.

Beyond the formal complaint processes, there is help on working through and understanding your feelings about your birth experience and information on birth trauma, stillbirth and neonatal loss. We are aware that men can suffer trauma after a birth too, so although the book is aimed at women much of the information and support applies to men as well. People and organisations for fathers to contact are listed in the Resources chapter.

The AIMS Guide to Resolution After Birth is also a handbook for those working in any part of maternity services, for birth workers and anyone supporting women and pregnant people through pregnancy, birth and beyond.

AIMS has recently published an Equality, Diversity and Inclusivity Statement which you can read at the front of this book. We understand that there is a huge diversity of people who use the maternity services and AIMS seeks to support all users.

How to get the best out of this book – an explanation of its structure

In the first chapter, Maria Booker helped me to explain which rights are protected by the Human Rights Act when accessing maternity services.

Chapter 2 is about 'consent' and an important one for everyone to read. Renew your understanding about what it means and how it feels to give consent in everyday life as well as for treatments or procedures.

Chapter 3 asks 'How do you feel?' You may need a pen and paper to work through this chapter as many questions are asked of you, and your answers form the basis for working through the issues, to help you understand your emotions or trauma.

Chapter 4 will help you to put your experience into some sort of context so that you can move forward and decide whether you should raise a concern or make a complaint.

Understanding birth trauma in Chapter 5, written by Dr Rebecca Moore, from Making Birth Better, describes the effects of devastating birth experiences.

Chapter 6 explains what to do if you or someone you know is referred to Children's Services. You might find it a bit shocking so please feel free to skip this chapter.

Chapter 7 is for those whose baby has died in childbirth, to help them to find resolution. This chapter was written for us by Clea Harmer from Sands.

Chapter 8 lists many of the people and organisations you can talk to for support.

Chapters 9 – 12 shows you how to work through the process of raising a concern or making a complaint.

Chapter 13 gives a brief overview of the Legal Action that can be taken in Maternity cases, and is written by Liz Thomas and Elizabeth Prochaska.

Chapters 14 and 15 help you prepare for a new pregnancy with where to go for support and help.

There is a useful Resources section at the back of the book.

Finally, we ask you to let us know how the guidance in this book works for you, so that we can understand your experiences of making complaints to the various organisations.

Language

AIMS understands that there is a huge diversity of people who use the maternity services. AIMS seeks to support all users, so we have tried to make the language in this book inclusive. Much of the time we use 'you' - directed at the reader who will usually be the maternity service user. We use the terms mothers or women when discussing research or guidelines in line with what the authors have used. Elsewhere we have used a mix of women, mothers, people, or pregnant women and people.

General Information

Guidelines are often referred to throughout the book. The professional bodies which regulate midwives and doctors are the Royal College of Midwives (RCM) and the Royal College of Obstetricians and Gynaecologists (RCOG) and they regularly publish guidance notes to aid good clinical practice. They do not dictate a single solution and the responsibility for your care still lies with the individual practitioner. You can find many examples of maternity guidelines on their websites *www.rcm.org.uk* (Blue Top Guidance) and *www.rcog. org.uk* (Green Top Guidance).

NICE (The National Institute for Health and Care Excellence) develop recommendations using the best available evidence to publish guidance in a number of areas – you might have heard of them in relation to their advice on the use of medicines. There are many guidelines about maternity care which can be found on their website *www.nice.org.uk*.

Finally, the book is packed full of information, and points the way to people and organisations who offer support. Remember that AIMS email and phone helplines are also there if you need them, *helpline@aims.org.uk* and +44 (0) 300 3650663. This phone number will connect you to an AIMS Volunteer when possible, otherwise please leave us a message, or email us, and someone will get back to you.

Chapter 1

Human Rights Law

The Human Rights Act incorporates the rights protected by the European Convention on Human Rights. The Convention sets out the minimum rights that all European Countries must respect. This means that if a person believes that their Convention rights have been violated, they can bring a legal claim in the UK courts. The Convention is not part of the European Union and it is anticipated that human rights protected by the Human Rights Act should not be affected by the UK leaving the EU because the UK will continue to belong to the Council of Europe.

Human rights in maternity care

Under the Human Rights Act 1998, pregnant women have the right to receive maternity care and to make their own choices about that care. The standard of care they are given must respect their dignity.

The Human Rights Act protects your dignity, privacy, equality and autonomy and requires all public bodies, including hospitals and Social Services, to treat pregnant women with dignity, to obtain their informed consent and to respect their decisions.

The UK has also ratified the Convention on the Elimination of Discrimination against Women. This prohibits pregnancy-related discrimination and requires the provision of healthcare for pregnant and lactating women.

What maternity rights are protected under the HRA?

Article 2 protects the right to life (of the woman, not the unborn child).

Article 3 sets out the right not to be subjected to inhuman or degrading treatment. There would be a violation of this article if a woman is neglected or treated in a way that is likely to cause serious harm or suffering when assessing and responding to the need for pain relief during and after childbirth, or when caring for women on postnatal wards, where they may be particularly vulnerable and require support for basic needs. The Mid-Staffordshire public inquiry revealed the impact that failure to respect basic dignity had on patients. The labour ward at Stafford Hospital was implicated in the scandal. Human rights claims brought under Article 3 on behalf of over 100 of the Mid-Staffs' patients have succeeded.

The Nursing and Midwifery Council, the professional regulator for nurses and midwives, is responsible for ensuring that professionals have the knowledge and skills to deliver consistent, quality care that keeps people safe. As a regulatory body, they take cases to court on patients' behalf, for example in Rostrom v. NMC (2009) it was found that '[The midwife] failed to uphold the dignity of a patient by allowing her to walk through the labour ward naked from the waist down and with a sanitary towel between her legs.'

Article 8 protects the right to respect for private and family life. Examples of violations could include not protecting the privacy of women during labour and on postnatal wards, not involving and supporting birth partners and not providing a translation to enable non-English speakers to make informed decisions about their care. The right to respect for private and family life is a qualified right; there are specific circumstances where it might be necessary to restrict it, for example to protect the rights of others or the needs of society. Any restriction must be lawful, serve a legitimate aim, and be necessary.

Article 8 was the focus of a case in 2014 where it was ruled that a local authority seeking to remove a child at birth must inform the mother of the care plan, except in exceptional circumstances (for example, if there is an immediate risk to the life of the newborn baby) Reference [2014] EWHC 3119 (Fam). Every mother facing a plan involving removal of her child has the right to be consulted and involved in that process, to protect her Article 8 rights (and those of the newborn baby). Another NMC case highlights this Article – Kostova v NMC (2013), a midwife was struck off the register for shouting at a patient 'you are no longer a human being but an animal.' The NMC found that she failed to respect the patient's dignity.

Article 9 protects the right to freedom of thought, conscience, and religion. As with Article 8, this is a qualified right and can be restricted in certain circumstances. Examples of potential violations may include not respecting a woman's choices based on her religious beliefs; for example she may have a preference for the gender of her health care professionals or a Jehovah's Witness may decline a blood transfusion even when the circumstances are life-threatening.

Finally, **Article 14** protects the right to enjoy these human rights without discrimination. It is a 'piggy-back' right because it must connect to the violation of another right. For example, if a midwife did not provide life-saving care (Article 2) based on a discriminatory attitude toward the woman based on her age or disability, gender or race, this would violate Article 14 as well as Article 2.

AIMS works closely with Birthrights, a charity dedicated to improving maternity care by promoting respect for human rights – *www.birthrights.org.uk* and Maria Booker, their Programmes Director, helped with the explanations above.

How AIMS works to protect and promote human rights in maternity care

» You will find the statement on human rights on the AIMS website[1]. The Human Rights Act underpins many of the rights you have and you will read more about it in this book to help you to understand its importance. Two articles in AIMS Journals[2,3] go into more depth about what this legislation means.

AIMS works with women on many issues that are covered by human rights legislation. These include:

- the provision of adequate maternity care
- the invasion of privacy
- coerced consent
- unnecessary or unexplained medical interventions
- a disregard of a woman's choice of
  - o how or where her birth takes place
  - o her birth partner
  - o her medical care giver
  - o her right for unassisted birth
- a lack of respect for women's dignity
- procedures carried out without consent.

---

1 *www.aims.org.uk/general/human-rights-law*

2 *www.aims.org.uk/journal/item/beyond-human-rights*

3 *www.aims.org.uk/journal/item/what-human-rights-legislation-means-for-aims*

These and many other situations may violate human rights and do lead to women being degraded and disempowered.

Issues for the LGBT+ community

There are many challenges faced by the LGBT+ community in maternity services for trans and non-binary people, not least that the law does not recognise some of their basic human rights in pregnancy and birth. For instance, when they register the birth of their child, they are not able to register themselves as their correct gender. A trans man who has given birth must be referred to on his child's birth certificate as the mother, when he might wish to be registered as the father. Stonewall's document 'A Vision for Change – Acceptance without exception for trans people 2017–2020'[4], gives clear information on this subject.

Acts such as the Equality Act 2010 state, 'a woman cannot be discriminated against for breastfeeding in public'. It is unclear whether the law would therefore protect a trans man, non-binary person or anyone else who is not a woman but is feeding their baby from their body, or if they would be treated differently for doing so. In order to safeguard their rights and claim their legal protection, they may have no option but to formally submit to being a woman, despite the distress that this may cause. Other rights, for instance, to body autonomy, and the right to make their own decisions, are not affected by LGBT+ status.

`

---

4 *www.stonewall.org.uk/system/files/a_vision_for_change.pdf*

Chapter 2

Consent

Although this book is about seeking resolution, most likely after giving birth, it is important to understand the concept of consent in its fullest sense. If you are reading this after something distressing has happened during your labour or birth, it may bring you more understanding; if you are reading this before giving birth, hopefully it will help you to prepare for any issues which may arise from your pregnancy or birth.

All medical procedures require our consent. This chapter is designed to make us think about the definition of consent and what it means for each of us. It will help us to understand how we consent, whether we are clear when we give consent and how we can withdraw consent. It will also help us to consider how we obtain consent from others and how it feels to give our consent.

Giving our consent is simple but can be complex at the same time. Simple in that we should be able to say 'yes' or 'no' and be respected for our decision. But complex because we are surrounded by social norms. For example, midwives and doctors are used to giving advice and it being followed – it's what they do every day and often without any issues – and so our consent may be assumed. There is a certain amount of indoctrination in the healthcare system (in any system anywhere).

You need to be concerned when the midwives and doctors just tell you what to do, or persuade you, maybe by providing misinformation, or persistently ask you when you have already said no, or threaten that terrible things will happen if you do not 'obey', when evidence or reality says otherwise. Coercing compliance to tests, assessments or procedures is not consent – and it is not just wrong and unethical, it is illegal.

The simplicity of consent

This definition on the NHS website[1] is very important. It states:

Consent to treatment is the principle that a person must give permission before they receive any type of medical treatment, test or examination.

- This must be done on the basis of an explanation by a clinician.

- Consent from a patient is needed regardless of the procedure, whether it's a physical examination, organ donation or something else.

- The principle of consent is an important part of medical ethics and international human rights law.

For consent to be valid it must be voluntary and informed, and the person consenting must have the capacity to make the decision:

- Voluntary – the decision to either consent or not to consent to treatment must be made by the person themselves, and must not be influenced by pressure from medical staff, friends or family.

- Informed – the person must be given all the information in terms of what the treatment involves, including the benefits and risks, whether there are reasonable alternative treatments, and what will happen if treatment does not go ahead.

---

1 *www.nhs.uk/conditions/consent-to-treatment/*

- capacity – the person must be capable of giving consent, which means they understand the information given to them and they can use it to make an informed decision.

The complexity of consent

Legally you have the right to decide, but in practice it is not always that straightforward. Midwives and doctors have routines in the care and treatment they provide. These can become second nature, part of their normal activity, and often they may forget or do not think to ask if you consent to what is being offered or done to you; this can become part of maternity practice culture. And it happens in life in general; people may come into your personal space and hug you; or people may touch a pregnant woman's belly as though it is public property! It may be a cultural issue but in Britain we would tend not to say anything. Perhaps you have your own ways of dealing with such situations. How do you deal with them?

When we are in hospital we can become compliant and inclined to submit to the authority of the midwives and doctors. The environment, equipment, staff and their uniforms can make us feel this way, so it is important for us to establish boundaries, however difficult that may be. Get into the habit of making conversation with them – what are you going to do, please explain it in full – and clearly state each time whether you agree – 'yes, you can do that' or you don't agree – 'no, you cannot do that'. It doesn't have to be with an aggressive tone – just remain calm and state your decisions. Many midwives and doctors will respect your decisions and work with you. Your birth plan is a crucial document to aid this purpose; it is important that your midwives and doctors know what is in it, so do not hesitate to make sure copies are available and ask them to read it.

A wider view of consent

Deciding whether to give your consent isn't just about saying yes or no. Our assumptions, expectations and feelings – such as pleasure, anger, unhappiness, fear – may be attached to our decision.

Although the following is from research about sexual consent and college students, the meaning of consent is further examined in an interesting and informative way. (1) From other research they note:

> " ... that the word consent can refer to a mental act (i.e. a decision or feeling of willingness) or to a physical act (a verbal or nonverbal expression of willingness)." (2)

The researchers talk about consent as an "internal state of willingness" – to wholly consent to what is offered the person must have willingness. The important thing is that this may not always be clear. How many times do we say "yes" just to be polite when we really mean "no"?

When we are offered medical care or treatment we need to be clear; we must give our 'explicit' consent. The midwife or doctor will ask us for verbal or written consent and we will give a precise and voluntary indication of our decision.

Implied consent is what someone else interprets as willingness. Consent is assumed because of a sign, an action, inaction, or even silence! An example of this is not saying anything when someone comes to hug us – whether we want them to or not.

One of the outcomes of the research found that women may soften their refusal to consent to avoid sounding arrogant or rude (remember the research is still in the context of sexual encounter) but we may find that this is quite a common way to refuse consent in British culture. To the person seeking consent, a softly spoken refusal may indicate a willingness to change one's mind – so they may try again. In this research, they found that some men saw a woman's refusal as something to overcome. This can happen in an interaction to obtain consent in a clinical setting where the person with the 'power' is the midwife or doctor who may see any refusal as something to overcome.

The research also mentions that consent can be a discrete, one-off event. For example, following a full discussion of the benefits and risks, you might be asked if you agree to a membrane sweep, an intervention where a midwife sweeps their finger around your cervix, with the aim and hope of releasing prostaglandin hormones to start labour. It is up to the them to obtain your informed consent for this; they can't legally do anything to you unless they have obtained your consent. It is a good example, because it is an intervention which you can agree to or not, or you can wait a while and think again.

> **If you reply** – **"Yes, you can do that"**. This means go ahead, I agree, I give consent.

> **If you reply** – **"No, you cannot do that"**. This is a clear statement of not giving consent. (Please note that it's not 'refusing to consent' either, which is another interpretation that midwives and doctors give to 'not giving consent'. If they write 'refused treatment' in your notes, ask that they reword it to read 'did not give consent'.)

> **If you reply** – **"No, not yet"**. With this reply you can make this into an ongoing, continuous process. I'm saying "no" now, but let's wait and see and I may agree later. You may ask me again.

If you don't have enough information to make a decision, you can ask as many questions as you like. One of the questions might be, "What are the pros and cons of waiting, or taking time to make a decision?" After asking the questions, in most cases you won't need to make a decision there and then.

Remember also that consent should be freely given and is reversible. You can always change your mind. The clearest way to do so is to say, "No, stop", but you might also say, "Stop, I don't like this" or "I need a break now". Once they have stopped doing whatever it is, you can take your time to explain what it is that you want to happen next. An extreme example of stopping a process would be during the preparation for a caesarean birth – you can't stop a caesarean birth once the incisions have been made but you can stop it right up to that point, even if you are in theatre and the team are ready to go. Some people have actually done this and whilst it is not easy, it is possible to do.

Acquiring knowledge

Your midwives and doctors should be skilled and knowledgeable, especially about up-to-date research information, so use their knowledge to help you to make the decision that you feel is right for you and your baby.

- You can ask them about the procedure, treatment or care they are offering AND the risks that may be present.
- You can ask if there are any alternative procedures or treatments that you can consider.
- You can also ask them "What if we do nothing?"

If you feel they are being one-sided

- you can ask more questions

  OR
- you can ask to be allocated another doctor or midwife.

You may wish to write notes on the discussion, or ask them to, or ask your birth partner to. You can also ask for a break so that you can have a think and talk to your birth partner and/or supporter, before you respond.

Hospital policy

If you are told that it is 'hospital policy', you can ask to read the policy and check the date that it was published. Many hospital policies are not up to date and not in line with national policy. Good places to look for national policy guidelines are RCOG (Royal College of Obstetricians and Gynaecologists) Green Top Guidelines[2], RCM (Royal College of Midwives) Blue Top Guidelines[3] and NICE (National Institute of Health and Care Excellence) Guidelines[4].

Guidelines should always have review dates and the interpretation and application of them is the responsibility of the doctors and midwives. The guidelines exist for the staff to know what you should be offered. You do not have to follow the guidelines if you don't want to! It is not the law. This is where your birth plan can come into its own – if you write it in advance of the birth you can find out the latest advice and decide what it is you would prefer. For example,

- you don't have to undergo vaginal examinations[5]
- the monitoring of your baby's heart rate in labour does not have to be done with an electronic fetal monitor (EFM)[6]
- your baby doesn't have to have a Vitamin K injection[7]
- you can choose whether you have pain relief[8].

---

2 *www.rcog.org.uk*

3 *www.rcm.org.uk*

4 *www.nice.org.uk*

5 *www.aims.org.uk/information/item/vaginal-examinations-in-labour*

6 *www.aims.org.uk/information/item/monitoring-your-babys-heartbeat-in-labour#post-heading-4*

7 *www.aims.org.uk/information/item/vitamin-k#post-heading-6*

8 *www.aims.org.uk/information/item/managing-labour*

Risks and benefits

How do you weigh up the risks and benefits of a medical procedure? If you are being asked your attitude to risk by a financial advisor, they might ask what you would do and how would you feel if you lost some or all of your money from a particular investment. It's fairly easy to answer this, and it will be based on whether you can really afford to lose the investment, your time frame, your need for return, etc. You will be given information about how the markets are performing and how the proposed investment has performed over time. You might compare the market to see which product will benefit you most.

In medicine, risks and benefits are a far more complicated subject because they affect your health and wellbeing and that of your baby. The terms 'risk' and 'benefit' refer to the outcome of a medical intervention. Evidence-based medicine will offer a benefit which you will then need to weigh up against the risks, or side-effects, associated with that intervention. It is important to discuss the risks and benefits with your midwife or doctor so that you completely understand the effects of any intervention or treatment that you are offered. Your thoughts about this are what matters, not those of the midwife and the doctor, as we all have different attitudes, fears and beliefs. Some questions you may wish to ask include:

- How big is the known risk of going ahead with this treatment?
- What are the side effects for me AND my baby?
- Please give me the benefits of treatment A compared to those of treatment B compared to doing nothing.
- How will my personal situation be affected by this treatment? e.g. will I be able to lift, drive, have sex etc.

The answers to risks may be quoted like this:

- 1 in 100 people benefit from this treatment.
- 4 in 1000 people will experience a side effect.
- 40 in 10,000 babies will have a better chance of ...

If you don't understand the above, ask your midwife or doctor to explain it to you in terms you do understand.

We have decisions to make and doing research into how risk is described and our own attitude to risk is important. You may wish to reflect on previous decisions you have taken – did you understand what the risks and benefits were? If the outcome was not as you hoped, was it because the risks or benefits were not properly explained? Or were the benefits of a procedure just not evident?

Empowerment

Do you feel empowered? This word is somewhat overused but it is useful in this context. You will know whether you feel empowered to make your decisions,

- if you have been given all the information about different options
- if you have been fully informed including all the pros and cons and possible outcomes of an intervention

    OR

    - you have been directed to all the relevant information
    - you have found it out for yourself

    AND you know that

- your decision will be based on what you want
- you have taken into account the risks
- you have listened to the opinions of experienced midwives and doctors and others

    OR

    - you are happy listening to your gut feeling.

Your midwives and doctors will respect your decision and support you 100%. This is the true outcome of informed consent and will give you that feeling of being empowered. You will feel in control.

Information has different dimensions, choices, risks and possibilities for each person – you are taking responsibility when you make a decision – you should feel powerful, empowered.

Again you may wish to reflect on previous decisions you have made. Did you feel comfortable with what you agreed? Were you given all the pros and cons and possible outcomes?

Safety

Treat any comments or advice raised by your midwives and doctors about safety as a consent issue, i.e. ask for the pros and cons and evidence, then decide what you want to do. Safety is important for you as well as for your baby. Sometimes an intervention may be recommended which might lead to a reduction in a very slight risk to your baby, but might lead to a significant increase in risk to you, in either physical or psychological ways. Safety in Childbirth (AIMS book) discusses the issues surrounding the safety of hospital birth, home birth and intervention free births.

How do you feel? Do you feel safe? Listen to your instincts. You matter, and you have the right to know what the possible outcomes are for your own long-term health and well-being, as well as those for your baby.

Parental responsibility – who can give consent for your baby

You, the mother, have the right to decide what happens to you and your unborn baby. You have the right to consent to treatment or not, even if the midwife or doctor thinks that your decision is putting you or your baby at risk of an adverse outcome, no matter what that might be. There doesn't have to be medical evidence to support your decision, neither do you need to justify your decision.

A question often asked is "can my partner or doula make decisions on my behalf" or "can I delegate my decision making?" The answer is that you should not want to delegate your decisions to someone else. They can support you in making your decisions, they can reiterate your decisions to the midwives and doctors, but they should not make your decisions for you. Similarly, a midwife or doctor cannot make decisions for you.

Your right to decide is enshrined in law in the UK. Only a judge in a court of law can rule that you are not able, i.e. that do not have 'legal capacity' according to very strict legal criteria, to make decisions for yourself about your body and unborn child. This is an extremely rare situation which is unlikely to occur when giving birth.

Obtaining consent during labour

Midwives and doctors have guidelines on how to obtain consent from women in labour. They are advised to discuss the person's preferred birth plan antenatally and to give you any relevant information or ask for your consent *between* contractions.

It is very helpful to have talked with your doctor or midwife about possibilities which might arise **before** you go into labour and to have your decision or preferred outcome documented in your birth plan. You might think about having an advocate (who knows your birthing preferences) with you when you are in labour, maybe a birthing partner or doula who can speak up for what you are saying you want or don't want, and if necessary raise the issue outside the labour room. Try to keep a note of the decisions you make, or ask a birth companion to do so, (your midwives and doctors should do this on your medical notes but your own copy might be something you find very helpful later).

The rights of the unborn and newborn baby

There is a difference between the unborn baby and the newborn baby in terms of rights in the UK. The unborn baby has no separate legal recognition and therefore does not have rights, whereas the newborn baby does (like any other child or adult). This means that in the interests of their unborn child as they see it, mothers have the right to consent to treatment or not. This may be different in other countries.

A mother automatically has parental responsibility for her child from birth. If the baby's father is married to the baby's mother, he usually has the same parental rights as the mother. The unmarried father may have parental responsibility too – if he has jointly registered the birth of the child with the mother, has a parental responsibility agreement with the mother, or has a parental responsibility order from the court.

Same-sex partners will both have parental responsibility if they were in a civil partnership at the time of treatment, i.e. donor insemination or fertility treatment. If the baby was created from sperm from a trans woman who is married to the baby's mother her rights are the same.

It is possible to have parental responsibility for the baby if you are not genetically related but more information about this is out of the scope of this book. In the absence of a court order, only those with parental responsibility can legally make decisions about what happens to the baby once it is born. For transgender people and those following a surrogacy path, we suggest seeking advice and support for your individual situation.

This information is very basic so if there is any uncertainty about your situation or a dispute arises it is best to seek professional advice. Each country, even within the United Kingdom, may have different rules, see *www.gov.uk/parental-rights-responsibilities/who-has-parental-responsibility*.

The people with parental responsibility give or decline consent to treatment and interventions on the baby's behalf. If the midwives and doctors disagree then the final decision may end up in court because treatment cannot go ahead unless permission is granted. However, in all circumstances it is hoped that some compromise and agreement can be reached early on in the discussions.

References

(1) Muehlenhard CL, Humphreys TP, Jozkowski KN and Peterson ZD, (2016) Complexities of Sexual Consent Among College Students: A Conceptual and Empirical Review. *e Journal of Sex Research*. 53:4-5, 457-487, DOI 10.1080/00224499.2016.1146651

(2) Beres, M. A. (2007) "Spontaneous' Sexual Consent: An Analysis of Sexual Consent Literature', *Feminism & Psychology*, 17(1), pp. 93–108. doi: 10.1177/0959353507072914.

Chapter 3

How do you feel?

We often go through a range of emotions after birth. If things didn't go as planned or healthcare workers were not being considerate or compassionate, our feelings are more complex. How do you feel about your birth experience now? It's important to write things down and if you are able to, to describe the time, the surroundings and intensity of feeling too. This will provide a great insight into what it was about the birth that made you feel the way you do as well as giving you a clue to the root causes of the feelings.

I will use the words 'upset' and 'complaint' to cover an array of feelings and the variety of concerns. There are many aspects to people's experiences and feelings, so when you are reading this book you might want to use the words that work best for **your** personal situation.

You may be screaming at the page, "I'm more than upset...." Or you might be thinking, "Well it's more of a concern....". You may feel irritated, violated, angry, or a whole range of mixed emotions after a birth and it might take some time to work out the cause or find words to describe them. The words displayed on the next page may help you.

angry

disappointed

shocked

scared

violated

helpless

overwhelmed

tearful

sad

confused

betrayed

robbed

not listened to

shamed

disconnected

lied to

relieved

disempowered

regretful

ignored

happy

thankful

broken

invisible

surprised

calm

content

peaceful

numb

hurt

upset

exhausted

guilty

lost

frustrated

grateful

If you feel able, one of the first and best actions to take is to write down how you feel and what you remember OR you might ask someone to do it for you or to help you do it. Make sure you are in an environment where you feel safe and comfortable, such as at home with someone around who you can call on, or in a cafe. You may prefer to be uninterrupted, in silence or with soothing music or white noise in the background. Write down your experience from beginning to end even if it is only in point form or phrases. Go back to it over several days when you feel able to. Take breaks if it feels too intense.

Repeat the process until you are satisfied you have written down everything you remember. This may include things like dates, times, names, (what the staff looked like if you do not recall their names), what was said to you, what actions staff took and when, how you felt and what you were thinking.

Once you have done that, highlight the areas which upset you the most, noting the timing and people present, and perhaps putting them in some sort of order, such as:

How you were treated e.g. not being listened to or respected.

The way you were spoken to or what was said to you.

The environment you were put in e.g. place of birth, privacy and dignity, lighting.

How your birth preferences were taken and supported.

Giving your consent/how you gave your consent.

How the way you were treated made you feel and still makes you feel, mentally and physically.

How the way you were treated affected your birth experience and outcome for you, your baby and family.

If there were specific people involved.

Was it one incident or a whole sequence or cascade of events?

Was it the consequences of an incident?

Were there aspects that were good?

Now put your complaint(s) under a main heading(s). Is it about:

how you were treated antenatally?

consent for treatment?

where you laboured and or gave birth?

how you were treated or spoken to when you were giving birth?

who was there when you gave birth?

how you were treated postnatally?

something other than the above?

It is a good idea to ask people (birth partners, doulas) who were with you to write down what they witnessed too.

Hopefully you will have a succinct description of what happened. The next chapter should help you to judge the sort of concern or complaint you may want to raise.

Chapter 4

Putting your experience into context and a recap of your rights

The subjects of the six words below are the main reasons for raising a concern or making a complaint about the experience you had during your pregnancy or birth.

It is just as important to read this chapter If you are pregnant now or planning to be pregnant, as knowing what to look out for will give you the opportunity to anticipate any problems which may arise and take action swiftly. It is important that we all increase our awareness of mistreatment, coercion and abuse in all it's possible forms. We know that making complaints will not solve all the problems but it's a start.

Consent

Mistreatment

Place of Birth

Your decisions

Discrimination

Medical Complications

Consent (*See Chapter 2*)

» You have to be given unbiased information and your **consent** must be obtained without influence or coercion for any treatment or intervention to be carried out legally – it is against the law for any midwife or doctor to do something to you for which you have not given consent. There are also guidelines about obtaining consent from women in labour if they are in pain or taking medication (*see also 'Obtaining consent during labour', p16*). The only exceptions to the law are when someone is considered not to have the capacity to make their own decisions or in an emergency situation, for example if you are unconscious.

» You should be given any information about tests, treatment or intervention for you AND your baby **before** anything is done. Giving consent does not have to be in writing – asking you to sign a document is more common for surgical procedures.

For example, a midwife should say to you, "Is it OK to give you an internal examination[1] in order to assess how far your labour has progressed?" She should explain to you that there are risks attached such as introducing infection, potentially stalling your labour and intensifying the pain you might be feeling. She should tell you that she will be able to judge your dilation for that moment of time, but that it will not tell you or her when the baby is coming. She should explain to you that she does not have to do it and that she has other skills at her disposal to make an assessment. You can say yes or no. If you say no, the midwife must accept that.

If she persistently asks after you have said no, you could take this as a warning sign and ask for another midwife.

---

1 *www.aims.org.uk/information/item/vaginal-examinations-in-labour*

Mistreatment (*see also Chapters 1, 12 and 13*)

It may be difficult to believe that you can be mistreated or abused in a UK hospital nowadays but it is possible and, very sadly, more common than you might expect. We are socialized to expect kind and professional care when we go to hospital for any reason and we are also likely to be compliant or at least try to be compliant. As a result there may be a power inequality and in this situation bullying and abuse may occur.

You have been mistreated, for example, if a midwife or doctor

- touched you without your consent
- shouted at you
- forced you to do something you didn't want to do
- forced you into a procedure you didn't want
- was rude to you or spoke to you unkindly
- made racist, sexist or degrading remarks
- did not allow you to do what you wanted or move how you wanted to
- denied you your choices
- deceived you, gave you misinformation or withheld important information
- sabotaged your birth
- restrained you when inappropriate to do so without explaining why
- denied you food or drinks during labour
- gave you medication without informed consent.

These examples are all abuses of your human rights; they may be against the law and they are most certainly in breach of professional codes of practice and conduct.

Place of birth

» You are legally entitled to make your own decision about where to give birth, even if you are deemed to be 'high risk'. You can choose to give birth at home or hospital. You cannot be compelled to give birth in a particular location or medical setting. Birth centres and hospitals will have admission criteria and you will be assessed. This will include your access to a birthing pool (*see p47, Professional Midwifery Advocate*).

» You can choose to have an unassisted birth, with no medical assistance at home – this is your legal right (*see p4*). If you do have a midwife present she must respect your decision. However, midwives and doctors may still believe you are placing your unborn child at risk, and they may tell you that they are going to make a referral to Children's Services (*see Chapter 6*).

Your decisions

» You can choose whoever you like to be at the birth. (*See Chapter 1*) However, there may be local rules in hospitals and birth centres about how many people you can have at the birth.

» If you request pain relief, you should receive it, unless there is a medical reason for withholding it or delaying it – your notes should explain if you didn't get it. Pain relief must not be withdrawn from you without asking for your consent. Withholding pain relief or delaying giving you pain relief must not be used to coerce you into compliance. For example, we hear from women that it is quite common to withhold pain relief until a vaginal examination is carried out (often on first reaching hospital). As explained in Chapter 2, Hospital policy (page 12) this is an example of exactly that and you don't have to consent to a vaginal examination.

Discrimination

The law protects you against discrimination, harassment and victimisation on grounds of age, disability, gender reassignment, pregnancy and maternity, race, religion or belief, sex and sexual orientation. Marriage and civil partnership status is also protected. These rights are enshrined in a law called the Public Sector Equality Duty 5 April 2011, created under the Equality Act 2010, relevant to England, Scotland and Wales.

Medical complications

You may be unwell during pregnancy, labour and the postnatal period because of a chronic disease such as heart disease, diabetes, or epilepsy, for example, or because of mental health issues which were diagnosed before your pregnancy. What you should experience because of your illness is enhanced maternal care (EMC) i.e. coordinated care across specialties targeted at your specific needs. Your midwives and doctors should know how to care for women and pregnant people with medical, surgical or obstetric problems during pregnancy, labour or in the postnatal period. For more information, please see the latest EMC guidelines published in August 2018 at *www.rcoa.ac.uk/ system/files/EMC-Guidelines2018.pdf.*

If any of the examples above or anything else that happened to you made you feel degraded or dehumanised and you felt that you were not given the care and respect that you are entitled to, these may be the 'cause for concern' or the basis for the complaint that you may wish to raise.

Staff may not have followed hospital policies or guidelines; they may have been unethical, unprofessional and/or negligent, your Human Rights may have been breached or the law may have been broken. Chapter 9 will take you further on your journey to raising a concern or making a complaint.

Chapter 5

Understanding birth trauma

By guest contributor, Dr Rebecca Moore, the cofounder of Making Birth
Better, *www.makebirthbetter.org. AIMS is a member of the Making Birth Better
network of parents and professionals which is dedicated to reducing the life-
changing impact of birth trauma.*

What is birth trauma?

Birth trauma describes a person's response to their birth experience if they
found one or more parts of that birth distressing, fearful or out of their
control. Birth trauma is common; studies estimate that 30–40% of women
find some part of their birth experience distressing. It's important to know
that birth trauma is not the same as postnatal Post-Traumatic Stress Disorder
(PTSD); a traumatic birth can lead to postnatal PTSD or you may have a
traumatic birth and not develop PTSD. Birth trauma can affect women and
men.

The things we have found distressing during birth are unique to us; it is
our birth and our individual experience. So, for some women this may have
been that they felt they were treated unkindly or that they were very alone
during birth, or that they felt staff ignored them or that they did not have
an opportunity to ask questions. For others, they may not have understood

what was happening because staff talked about them not to them. Or it may be that something happened medically that made a woman feel they were at risk of serious harm or even of dying or that their baby might die. For some women, birth can feel like an assault or that they were coerced or bullied into procedures or decisions that they did not consent to or understand.

Women can have a range of responses to birth trauma, which can last for weeks, months or even years. They may go on to develop depression, with a persistent sense of low mood or sadness, a loss of enjoyment in life and fatigue and tiredness with altered sleep and appetite and sometimes suicidal ideas.

Women can develop Obsessive Compulsive Disorder (OCD) after birth trauma, this may mean recurrent intrusive obsessional thoughts about safety or harm, these fill the mind constantly and make thinking about anything else seem hard, these thoughts feel out of control and may loop round and round in one's head. Compulsions are behaviours that develop to try to feel in control or reduce anxiety, this might be checking the doors or windows or the baby or cleaning the house in a certain order.

PTSD involves reliving your birth repeatedly in your mind with thoughts or in your dreams as nightmares, feeling constantly on edge and alert and scanning for risk, avoiding things that remind you of your trauma, thinking about your birth, talking about your birth, pregnant friends, hospitals, sex or even your baby along with disturbed sleep, appetite and concentration.

Some women can be very traumatised by birth without any symptoms of a clinical illness, yet the experience can have a huge effect on their daily lives, especially as they start the journey into motherhood. Women can feel unable to connect with their baby or that they cannot let their baby out of sight in case something bad happens. Their sexual relationship can be affected too and they may feel irritable or resentful towards their partner and family for failing to help or protect them.

Women can experience many feelings due to birth trauma; they may seem completely preoccupied with their birth, replaying it in their mind and talking about it incessantly, or they may avoid talking about it or seeing pregnant friends or even going anywhere near the hospital where they gave birth. They will often have nightmares or disturbed sleep and wake up feeling exhausted and persistently on edge and worried that something bad may happen to them or their baby.

Anyone in the birth room can be traumatised and we know that birth partners are often affected as well as staff working in the maternity setting. It can be very frightening for fathers and partners because they are able to watch everything that is happening but may feel powerless to help and very separate from what is going on.

What may help?

We know that birth trauma is not easily recognised, and people are often told they are depressed when they are not. GPs and health visitors are not good at diagnosing birth trauma or PTSD; some are, of course, but not all. Many women are never given the time and space to fully describe their birth experience.

We have some free crib sheets on *www.makebirthbetter.org/cribsheets* that people can download to take to their GP to show them the symptoms they are having to help make the correct diagnosis. Broadly, with depression we would look for a low mood all the time, whereas after trauma moods tend to be up and down; with depression we look for a complete loss of enjoyment in life and with trauma this is not so common. In depression we would not expect to see a recurring reliving of the birth experience with nightmares or disturbing dreams, as this is more typical of birth trauma. The key is to see an expert who you can talk to about how you are feeling; this can seem very hard, but you might have a good GP already or a good health visitor. Ask to see your local perinatal champion GP if you can or speak to a helpline such as PANDAS[1], *www.pandasfoundation.org.uk* or AIMS, *www.aims.org.uk.*

Many women with birth trauma ask for a hospital debrief. The quality of these debriefs is mixed and very much depends on who does the debrief and how. Make sure you take someone with you for support; and know that you are allowed to take notes and/or to record the debrief session. For many women, it can be simply too painful to go back to the maternity department where their trauma took place, or the debrief can feel more like a meeting where the Trust tries to make sure that a legal claim is not pursued. If the staff and the hospital trust are defensive and determined to dismiss any information that they fear might lead to a legal claim, this can make trauma, anxiety and PTSD symptoms worse.

However, if the staff facilitating the session are being open and honest and willing to acknowledge the mother's experience, a debrief can be very helpful because you will understand the sequence of events of the birth and be able to ask questions about the interventions that were used and why.

Some women go on to make a formal complaint and benefit from feeling that they told the Trust how they felt. They feel that they may have influenced a change in some of the practices; some women go back to teach and train staff locally or become passionate campaigners or peer supporters.

Formal treatments

There are many treatments for birth trauma, but they are not always available locally and many women end up sourcing treatments privately, which can be a huge financial pressure.

---

1 *PANDAS Foundation UK is a support service for families suffering prenatal, ante-natal and postnatal illnesses which has a free daily helpline and email support.*

Treatments can include exercise, supplements, peer support, journaling, online social media support, scar massage, tapping, somatic work or therapy, physiotherapy, trauma focused CBT therapy or EMDR, meditation and/or medication. In many areas you can now self-refer for counselling by contacting your GP's surgery or local mental health teams. Not all of these teams are specialists in treating trauma so there can be long waits to access treatment and there may be a waiting list.

If you are looking for a therapist, look for someone who can offer trauma-focused Cognitive Behaviour Therapy (TF-CBT) or Eye Movement Desensitisation Reprocessing (EMDR). My colleague, Emma Svanberg, has written an article for the *AIMS Journal* which goes into more detail about the therapies for birth trauma, *www.aims.org.uk/journal/item/cbt-emdr*. Her book *Why Birth Trauma Matters* is available now from Pinter and Martin booksellers.

TF-CBT involves helping individuals to make sense of their experiences, identify ways or patterns of thinking that are negative, recognise these thoughts and beliefs about them self, others or the world associated with the traumatic event, and note their behavioural or coping responses.

EMDR (Eye Movement Desensitization and Reprocessing) is a therapy that uses eye movements (or other bilateral stimulation) during one part of the session. After the clinician has determined which memory to target first, they ask the client to hold different aspects of that event or thought in mind and to use their eyes to track the therapist's hand as it moves back and forth across the client's field of vision. As this happens the clients begin to process the traumatic memory.

Private therapists typically charge £50–150 per session. You can find therapists through the British Psychological Society (BPS) (*www.bps.org.uk*) and/or the British Association for Counselling and Psychotherapy (BACP) (*www.bacp.co.uk*).

Conclusion

In this article I have described birth trauma and highlighted some of the reasons for women being traumatised by their birthing experience. I have suggested various ways that you may seek help and I urge you to take those first steps – there are people who can and will help you. There are gentle ways to seek resolution as well as following a more formal route. Healing and recovery are possible with time, kindness and specialist support.

Chapter 6

Fear of referral to Children's Services

Safeguarding and Child Protection

Whilst it is parents and carers who have primary care for their children, local authorities working with partner organisations have specific duties to safeguard and promote the welfare of all children in their area. The Children Act 1989 puts a duty on the local authority to provide services to children in need in their area. The same Act requires local authorities to undertake enquiries if they believe a child is at risk of significant harm.

Everyone who works with children and families (for example, in health, the police, in education and in social care and housing) has a role to play in safeguarding and promoting the welfare of children which is defined as:

- Protecting children from maltreatment.

- Preventing impairment of children's health or development.

- Ensuring that children grow up in circumstances consistent with the provision of safe and effective care.

- Taking action to enable all children to have the best outcomes[1].

1 Working Together to Safeguard Children 2018, *https://assets.publishing.service. gov.uk/government/uploads/system/uploads/attachment_data/file/779401/Working_Together_to_Safeguard-Children.pdf*

Social Services run Children's Services and Adult Social Care. Safeguarding children is the term used to cover the descriptions in the above list and include preventative measures to keep children healthy and safe. Child Protection is a single aspect of safeguarding, one which focuses on protecting a child who is suffering or has the potential to suffer significant harm. A Child Protection referral will inevitably lead to an assessment by a social worker.

What is a referral?

A referral to Children's Services is when somebody, e.g. a parent, teacher, neighbour, midwife, doctor (anyone can make the referral), contacts the local authority because they have concerns about the safety or well-being of the child. On the whole referrals are made with the best interest of the family at heart but some people, including midwives and doctors, have a limited understanding of what warrants a referral to social care and so many unnecessary referrals are made. AIMS hears from women who have been threatened with a referral by a midwife or doctor as a way to coerce them into agreeing care or treatment that they are reluctant to have. This is unacceptable and can be reported through the appropriate channels within the hospital.

Where to get help?

It can be incredibly distressing to discover that a referral has been made about you and your family, but it is important that you engage with Children's Services as usually unfounded or unnecessary referrals can be sorted out quickly during your initial meeting with a social worker.

Women tell us that seeking help and advice quickly is crucial, and we know that individual Children's Services can vary greatly. The Family Rights Group (*www.frg.org.uk*) is the charity in England and Wales which can provide the support and information people need and advise you about your rights and options when social workers or courts are about to make decisions about your child or unborn baby. Their advice line 0808 801 0366 is open Monday to Friday 9.30–3.00. Their website is full of vital information *www.frg.org.uk* including fact sheets, FAQs, films explaining the child welfare system, and discussion boards where you can ask questions and 'talk' to their adviser and other parents. They also have a range of advice sheets which can be downloaded for free: *www.frg.org.uk/ need-help-or-advice/ advice-sheets.*

You can request a family support worker by contacting your local Children's Centre. The family support worker is there to help families who are experiencing short- or long-term difficulties, maybe with long term health problems, mental health problems, financial or marital issues, language, or drug or alcohol addiction. They will have qualifications in the care of children and in safeguarding, and will come from a variety of backgrounds such as childcare, community work, counselling, education, youth work and social care. They will be employed by the local authority or by charities.

Citizens Advice, *www.citizensadvice.org.uk*, may be able to help you too. They should be able to talk you through your rights and what might happen, and they will also be able to give you a list of local solicitors. Be aware that in any given town some solicitors will act for Children's Services, and others specialise in advocating for the parents so it is important to ask who they act for, as there may be a conflict of interest.

Civil Legal Advice is a free and confidential service run on behalf of the government for England and Wales. They may help you to work out if you are entitled to free legal advice and again help you to find a solicitor – telephone them on 0345 345 4345 Monday to Friday 9am to 8pm, Saturday 9–12.30pm. Their website is *www.gov.uk/ civil-legal-advice.* They have a free call back service. You will need to provide copies of recent payslips, bank statements, details of any savings or investments, details of any benefits and mortgage statements.

AIMS can provide information and support in relation to maternity issues and rights, information which may be important for you in relation to challenging the basis of a referral. Our volunteers on AIMS helpline can provide information and listen during this stressful time, but cannot be involved in individual cases. Unfortunately, AIMS do not have the resources, either in time or experience to be of practical help if you are referred to Children's Services.

There are two assessments used by social workers that you should know about. These are:

Pre-birth Assessment

If you are referred to Children's Services or already have children who are not in your care, you may be required to have a pre-birth assessment. This entails the social worker asking you about yourself, the baby's father, your relationship status, your home, your employment status, your financial situation and what support you have. The social worker will then make an assessment to see if you can meet the baby's needs – it will be an in-depth and usually constructive discussion.

Be as honest and open as possible, but keep notes about what you say, and do as much preparation and research into the process as possible yourself. Think of the positives, for things in your favour; if you already have a child in care, try to share any insight you have into why it happened that time. Be very clear to them about the support you have from your family and friends. The social workers will want to see the baby's father as well, if possible.

It is very important to stay calm and not get angry. It is common for parents to feel threatened or cornered in these situations which can aggravate anger, but they will be looking to see how you behave. Some women have told us that their reactions were interpreted as hostile and were used against them. If you feel it is starting to become overwhelming, ask for a short break so that you can have a drink of water, digest the information and gather your thoughts, then continue the conversation.

Following this assessment, the social workers may arrange a child protection conference whilst you are still pregnant; this is to make sure your baby is kept safe after it is born. You should be invited to attend this meeting and be allowed to take a supporter or advocate with you.

Always ask what Children's Services plans are for your baby after birth, including whether and when you will be required to go to court.

Viability Assessment

This is to assess whether any of your family or friends can take care of your baby; this is known as kinship care. Other people have had brothers or sisters who have been able to volunteer in this way. If your parents could be possible volunteers, this website may prove helpful *www.grandparentsplus.org.uk*.

When things go wrong

Many social workers are dedicated and caring people doing their best to help the children and families they are working with, often in difficult circumstances. Unfortunately, there are times when this is not always the case.

- You are entitled to request a support person of your choice to be present at meetings and visits and we hear from women on AIMS helpline that it is really important to have someone with you.

- You can apply for access to all records held about you under the General Data Protection Regulation (GDPR). The link to the Information Commissioner's Office website is *ico.org.uk/your-data-matters/* and see Chapter 12, page 78 for more information.

- Social workers will ask you for your permission to access your (and those of any children and your baby's) health records; you have the right to refuse, but if there is a significant cause to suspect any child or children is suffering or is likely to suffer significant harm, they can request them direct from the hospital or GP Surgery.

- You can ask for a different social worker, but you do not have a right to demand a change, so it may not happen.

- The Family Rights Group may be able to provide professional advocacy to parents.

- You may be able to have an advocate at your meetings or hearings – ask your social worker if they can arrange it.

- You can take notes during the meeting, as can your supporter.

- You can ask to record conversations and meetings – explain that you have trouble remembering what was said and that this would help your understanding.

- Always send any letters to Children's Services by registered mail.

- You may also consider looking for some mental health support as many find this a stressful experience. AIMS acknowledges the threat or potential threat of separation of mother and baby can lead to unknown trauma for both, and needs to be explicitly addressed in the safeguarding procedures.

- You may be able to complain, but discuss it with the Family Rights Group advice service first, as the complaints procedures are focused on child welfare.

Because the law and procedures are very complicated AIMS is unable to provide further information and support. However, we would always recommend:
- to always have someone else with you,
- to make notes about any conversations you have,
- to obtain advice from a knowledgeable person as soon as possible.

Light at the end of the tunnel

It has been reported in the Law Society Gazette 11 December 2019[2] that new guidelines will be developed in the coming months to acknowledge the issues surrounding care proceedings for newborns. The report says: 'Given the vulnerability of infants and their mothers in the immediate post-natal period, issuing care proceedings at or close to birth is fraught with moral, ethical and legal challenges – and without effective, timely assessment and support during pregnancy, intervention at birth is likely to be poorly planned and can result in instability for the new baby and huge distress for family members.' To read the report, go to *www.nuffieldfjo.org.uk/resource/pre-birth-assessment-and-infant-removal-at-birth-experiences-and-challenges.*

Give this information to family and friends, as well as social workers and the midwives and doctors to give them an understanding of the issues.

---

2 *www.lawgazette.co.uk/practice/guidelines-for-judges-to-divert-newborns-from-care-proceedings/5102465.article*

Chapter 7

Why did my baby die?

By guest contributor Clea Harmer, Chief Executive of Sands (Stillbirth and Neonatal Death Society). She would like parents to receive the correct bereavement care and understand why their baby died.

Tragically, every year in the UK over five thousand babies die before, during or shortly after birth. In 2017, 3,200 babies were stillborn (babies who died after 24 weeks' gestation but before they were born) and there were 2,131 neonatal deaths (babies who died in the first 4 weeks of life).

We are so sorry if you are reading this and your baby has died. Nothing can take away the pain and devastation of the death of your baby, but it is important to know that you are not alone and there are many places to find support and further information – see *www.sands.org.uk/usefullinks*.

Straight after your baby has died it is often hard to think through what you might need or want. The healthcare professionals looking after you should give you the bereavement care you most need at this time, helping you to make memories of your baby, make decisions about funerals and about post mortems, and giving you the time and space you need to be with your baby.

One of the most important things is to understand *why* your baby died; this is an essential part of grieving for your baby and your baby's 'story', but it is also necessary to understand if anything went wrong and, if it did, to identify what must be learned to prevent the same thing happening to other babies and families. It is also crucial to know if there is anything that might affect your decisions in future pregnancies and births.

Not all baby deaths are understood and more research is needed into why some babies die. However, there are two processes that might help provide answers; the first of these is a post mortem, which is a clinical investigation to understand any factors that might have contributed to your baby's death and is undertaken by a specialist pathologist. You should be offered the chance to have a post mortem on your baby but not every family will feel this is the right option for them. It is vital that parents are supported to make decisions that are right for them and their baby. This parent to parent post mortem film may be helpful, *https://sands-lothians.org.uk/post-mortem-animation/*.

Another process that helps to provide answers is a review or investigation, which should be carried out to make sure that what happened is fully understood and lessons can be learned. There are several different types of review or investigation: all babies who die after 22 weeks gestation in the UK are reviewed using the Perinatal Mortality Review Tool (PMRT); for those deaths where something may have gone wrong, further NHS Serious Incident Investigations are undertaken by the Trust or Health Board; in England, stillbirths that happen at the end of pregnancy are investigated by the Healthcare Safety Investigation Branch; the Child Death Overview Panel reviews all neonatal deaths. More information on reviews can be found at *www.sands.org.uk/support-you/understanding-why-your-baby-died*.

In all these reviews and investigations, you should be given the opportunity to be involved in a way that feels comfortable for you – this will allow you to share your perspective and any information you have that you feel might be relevant. You should be kept informed about the review throughout the process – remember to ask who will do this for you.

Currently, a coroner (procurator fiscal in Scotland) will usually only be involved if the baby has died after birth (neonatally) and may open an inquest if there is concern about the circumstances of the death. The involvement of the coroner or procurator fiscal can provide a further opportunity to understand why a baby might have died, though if the reviews or investigations have been completed well the answers may already be known. An inquest may provide answers but can take 6 to 12 months to complete.

Bereaved parents often say that they want to make sure that no other parent goes through what they have been through. Using reviews and investigations to understand what happened every time a baby tragically dies is an important way to make sure that real learning happens, and that any necessary changes are made.

Practical Steps to a Resolution

The following diagram maps some of your options after a bad maternity experience. There are clear routes to follow, but discussing your experience with one of the people suggested in the following chapter is a good place to start.

The chapters following give a comprehensive summary of the different avenues open to you. It depends on what you want to achieve: Do you want to complain or just raise a concern? Do you want an apology or financial compensation? Do you want things to change so no-one else has to experience what you experienced? Do you want to find help? These options, and many more, are discussed in the book, as well as how to access the agencies or people that you would like to contact.

Whichever route you take, we advise you to obtain your maternity notes first (*see Chapter 10*).

Practical steps to resolution after a bad maternity experience

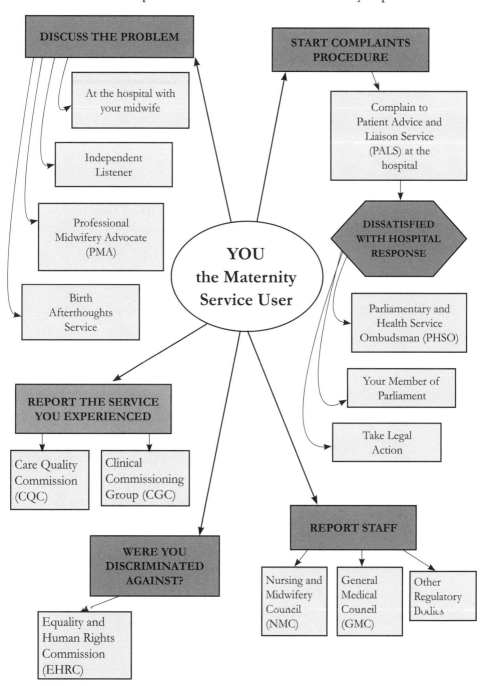

Chapter 8

People or organisations you can talk to

Listed in this chapter are a number of specialist people or organisations where you may be able to get support, help or advice. It is important that you consider who best to approach – the options are laid out for you, but what is right for one person may not be right for another.

How you are feeling may give you some idea of whom you want to meet with and whether you want to meet anyone from the hospital where you gave birth. Think about who can go with you as we would not recommend going by yourself. It's a good idea to take someone because then there is someone else to listen and perhaps write down what is said for you. They may even be able to give you a different perspective or pick up on different things. If it's you and your partner then you can always ask to take a third person in to listen and take notes. You can also ask to record the session.

You may well feel that these services are too threatening for you. You may have concerns which you do not wish to share with the people whom you feel may have caused the problems. In this case, it is important that you find support away from the health service establishment where it happened.

Please be clear that the list is simply that – we do not have the knowledge and experience to rate or advise on any of these services, and they may well be very different depending on where you live and they may change over time.

From the hospital or community

The Professional Midwifery Advocate (PMA) or if your hospital does not yet have one, a consultant midwife or the Head of Midwifery should be able to help you. The PMA has been or hopefully will be established in each hospital under the A-Equip model. This is a new role which replaced Supervisors of Midwives (SOMs), but is not available everywhere yet. PMAs are senior midwives with a special role:

- to give guidance and support to both you and your midwife
- to ensure your care is appropriate and delivered in the right place, by the right person and that it will benefit you and your baby
- to help midwives to access additional education and training in practice as necessary

and a PMA can support you

- by listening and advocating on concerns you may have about your current midwifery care
- by talking to your midwife/obstetrician on your behalf if you are concerned about your plan of care
- by supporting and advising on care choices, such as place of birth
- by enabling good communication between you and your midwife in relation to your care.

You may request a meeting with **your consultant obstetrician or your midwife**. Alternatively, you may ask to see a different Consultant Obstetrician or the Head of Midwifery. They should be able to discuss your individual case with you and help you to understand what happened.

You can request a meeting with the **PALS service** (Patient Advice and Liaison Service) – they provide a free, confidential service offering support to help you sort out any concerns you may have and to guide you through the different services provided by the Trust.

There may be a **Birth Afterthoughts Service** in your hospital (ask your midwife, GP or health visitor). You can meet (either in the hospital or at home) with a specially trained midwife, who will go through your labour and birth notes explaining in some detail what happened and answer your questions. She should be able to tell you whether things were avoidable or unavoidable and be able to refer you for counselling, if necessary or if you request it. This meeting can take place at the hospital or another place of your choice.

We have feedback which gives mixed views about the quality of these afterbirth services. A recent report[1] found provision was limited both in numbers of hospitals which have the service and in the quality of the service itself. Many of the services were provided by midwives who had no specialist training and whilst there was flexible access to the services, discussions centred on birth trauma were less evident. Women tell us that staff who carry out the debriefing at the hospital may be defensive and that, naturally, can make the woman feel even worse.

AIMS suggests that you try and find out from other women locally whether the service in your hospital is a good one. This is a situation where personal recommendation could be the key to your decision. If this proves impossible, it is better to go forewarned that the meeting might not meet your expectations and/or needs. If this is the case, you can just leave the meeting at any time.

---

1 Gill Thomson, Charlotte Garrett, 'Afterbirth support provision for women following a traumatic/distressing birth–: Survey of NHS hospital trusts in England, *Midwifery* (2019), doi: *https://doi.org/10.1016/j.midw.2019.01.004 1*

These services give hospitals a chance to resolve your queries, which may otherwise escalate into a complaint. However, if you are not satisfied with what you have been told you still have the option to make a complaint.

Independent listeners

Independent midwife or doula

Something many women have found helpful is having an informal discussion or birth review with an independent midwife; she may be able to explain what happened and you can go through your maternity notes or ask questions at your own pace. There is usually a small fee for this service. You can find a list of Independent Midwives on the website, *www.imuk.org.uk*. If you had a **doula**, she may be able to help you understand what happened, and give you her recollections and reflections.

Your GP Surgery

A **GP** should be able to provide a listening ear and perhaps refer you for counselling or to the **Perinatal Mental Health Team** (there will probably be a long wait for this service). It is worth asking if there is a 'birth trauma' pathway so you can be fast tracked to access psychotherapy.

For your physical healing, there may be a **physiotherapist** specialised in rehabilitation of the pelvic floor and resolving incontinence symptoms. If they are not on-site at your surgery, you can ask to be referred to a place of your choice such as the Women's Health Clinic at your local or another Trust. Physiotherapy is about working with your body. Some GPs may recommend an appointment with a gynaecologist and you can decide whether you would like to go ahead or try the physiotherapy exercises first. Keep in mind gynaecology tends to be more focused on surgery.

Local Organisations

The local **National Childbirth Trust** (NCT) may have someone you can speak with who has had a similar experience. Your local NCT branch is a good source of information about other local groups. Your health visitor may also be able to help you.

National Organisations

Action against Medical Accidents (AvMA)

AvMA is a UK charity which provides free independent advice and support to people affected by medical accidents ('lapses in patient safety'). Their website is extremely useful; it has self-help guides about the complaints procedures, you can request support at inquests and ask about possible legal action. They also have information about claims for birth injuries both for the baby and the mother. For more information, visit their website at *www.avma.org.uk/help-advice/*.

Healthwatch

You can contact your local Healthwatch to find out how to get help with making your complaint or go to their website *www.healthwatch.co.uk* search > Help making a complaint. The pages eventually take you through to Citizens Advice – these website pages are helpful.

Maternity Transformation Programme

Campaigning is often a good way to change a service and healthcare culture. If you would like to be involved, consider joining a Maternity Voices Partnership(MVP) or any of AIMS' campaigns.

Better Births[2] is the report of the National Maternity Review, published in February 2016, setting out a clear vision of maternity services across England.

The Maternity Transformation Programme has been set up to drive and oversee the process of delivering the recommendations of the report and has spawned the Local Maternity Systems (LMS) and Sustainability and Transformation Plans (STPs). Each LMS must have a clear STP, involving all local commissioners and providers as well as service user forums, by 2020/21. The LMS must encourage service-user participation and co-production[3].

MVPs are being set up and comprise a team of women, their families, commissioners and providers (midwives and doctors) working together to review and contribute to the development of local maternity care.

If you want to campaign to change things, it will be worth contacting your local Maternity Voices Partnership or you can even set one up in your area if it

2 *www.england.nhs.uk/wp-content/uploads/2016/02/national-maternity-review-report.pdf*

3 There is not one definition of co-production that everyone agrees on because the approach is still developing and changing. The New Economics Foundation, NEF, suggests co-production is 'The relationship where professionals and citizens share power to design, plan, assess and deliver support together. It recognises that everyone has a vital contribution to make in order to improve quality of life for people and communities'. See also, *www.thinklocalactpersonal.org.uk/co-production-in-commissioning-tool/co-production/In-more-detail/what-is-co-production/*

doesn't already exist! Details are on the website *http://nationalmaternityvoices. org.uk/wp-content/uploads/2017/11/Better-Births-resource-pack-for-LMS-asummary-for-MVPs-v1.pdf* and please see *AIMS Journal* 30/1[4] and 30/2[5] Better Births 1 and 2, for more information.

Board Level Champion

In the Better Births report, under the section headed Safer Care, there is an interesting idea that each 'provider board' (your local hospital has a trust board) should have a board level champion for maternity services. The 'champion' should be routinely monitoring information about quality, including safety, and take necessary action. AIMS suggests that you contact this person in writing about your concerns, but as it is a new idea we do not have any reports of people's experiences.

Social Media

If you like searching online for information, be careful. Make sure you know that the people behind the page are reputable, and check your privacy settings. It is best not to post any private information. If the comments on the page are rude, negative or generally upsetting, withdraw from the site. It is better to find a real person to talk to! Contact the AIMS helpline or your midwife or therapist.

---

4 *www.aims.org.uk/journal/index/30/1*

5 *www.aims.org.uk/journal/index/30/2*

Chapter 9

Whether to raise a concern or make a formal complaint?

You have a right to raise a concern (tell the staff what went wrong so that hopefully they will not make the same mistake again) or make a formal complaint. This chapter is intended to help you decide by answering the questions posed.

Think about what would you like the outcome to be or what would you like to achieve? Would you like:-

- an acknowledgement of what happened
- an apology stating that you should not have been treated in the way you were treated
- an explanation
- a change to hospital policy
- to stop what happened to you from happening to someone else
- a member(s) of staff to understand how their actions have affected you
- compensation
- remedial treatments for yourself and/or your baby
- to alert the authorities of dangerous practices or hospital cultural issues
- something else.

The following questions may help you to reflect on your situation if your concern or complaint is about a member of staff.

- Do you think there was an intention to cause harm (physically or mentally)?

- Did they listen to and respect you?

- Do you think the member of staff was unwell or tired?

- Do you think there were not enough staff on duty?

- Were they following protocols instead of consulting with you and keeping you informed of what was happening?

- Have you or has someone you know been in a similar situation before, but where you or they were treated differently?

- You might not be aware of the procedure, or process or guideline, but do you think there might be one covering the complaint you are making? For example, if the complaint is about how the member of staff spoke to you, do you know if they are subject to guidelines about that?

Write down your reasons and reflect on them for a little while, and hopefully this will give you clarity on what action to take and which aspects to focus on.

What will happen if you raise a concern?

If you raise a concern, it is likely to be a one-way communication. You can say what you need to and send it to whoever you want to read it – it gets it 'off your chest' and 'out of your head'. You will need to have low expectations of receiving a reply, because you are not in a formal system. However, you might be surprised and receive a positive answer!

What will happen if you make a formal complaint?

Making a formal complaint is not for the fainthearted and there are no guarantees that you will get the outcome you are looking for. However, if you do not complain the opportunity to change or improve something may be lost.

In making a formal complaint, you should gain understanding and perhaps put pressure on your local maternity or healthcare system to change. People may choose not to complain about their treatment or what happened to them and their babies in childbirth for various reasons, but it may be part of your own healing process to pursue a formal complaint. On the other hand, you might feel your recovery would be damaged by making a complaint. However, it is a chance to speak up, to seek acknowledgement and maybe even receive an apology for what has happened.

For a view of how the management of the Trust concerned may examine your complaint, please refer to 'A Just Culture Guide – supporting consistent, constructive and fair evaluation of the actions of staff involved in patient safety issues' at *https://improvement.nhs.uk/documents/2490/NHS_0690_IC_A5_web_version.pdf*.

Once you have answered all the questions raised in this section, you may have come to a decision. You may decide to raise a concern that you have identified, in which case you can write it down and send your feedback to the Director of Midwifery or somebody else you identify, explaining that you don't need a response, just an acknowledgement of receipt. You can also tell the Care Quality Commission #Declareyourcare (*see page 75*). However, if you decide to make a formal complaint there is advice in the following chapters to help you.

Chapter 10

Obtaining your health records

Before you decide exactly what your options are, it is probably a good idea that you obtain a copy of your health records, sometimes referred to as case notes, and your maternity hand held notes – this is a FREE service.

You may have your own set of 'hand held' medical records known as maternity notes which you should have been given at your first antenatal appointment for use throughout the pregnancy. However, there will be another set of records completed by the midwives and doctors, inevitably during labour and the birth but perhaps at other times too. Some hospitals are starting to have on-line records too. *Which?*, the consumer watchdog, have a section on their website for all things birthing. In particular they have good information about what your health notes mean[1].

You have the right to see and receive a copy of all your health records, and those of your baby – the records will include written notes, any computerised records, and any additional letters or memos. You do not need a reason to ask for them. You need to apply to the organisation responsible, either your GP surgery or the Medical Records Manager at your hospital – you can usually

---

1 *www.which.co.uk. Search > Scans, appointments and classes*

do this online. You may have to fill in an application form and give proof of your identity, and make a separate application for your baby.

If you cannot do it online and there is no form, apply in writing giving your full name, date of birth, NHS number (if you know it), address, telephone number and which records you wish to see, e.g. your recent stay (with dates) in the Maternity Unit. It is recommended that you keep a copy of your letter and send it by Signed For: Proof of Delivery via the Post Office. You should receive copies of the records within one month of requesting them.

Sometimes the photocopies are indistinct and it is worthwhile checking exactly what is written. You can also check that the times and dates are clear, as these are often near the edge of the pages and it is not uncommon for them not to appear on the photocopy. If you have any cause to suspect that they may not be accurate, you can arrange to go into the hospital to see the originals of the health records. Also, the original notes will show where there has been an alteration or an addition – photocopies may not reveal that. Ask for this viewing to take place in the Medical Records Department of the hospital with administration staff. It is wise not to make any comments about the notes during the viewing – keep your comments for any letter you may wish to write later.

If your issue involves previous obstetric or gynaecological experiences that may have occurred in other hospitals, you should apply for your health records at the other hospitals too. Likewise, if your issue involves your health visitor, GP, private care, or social workers, you can apply for their records about you and your baby.

You can ask questions of the volunteers on the AIMS Helplines. Although we do not have the resources to help you with an in-depth case we can signpost you to the right people.

Please note also:

- AIMS recommends obtaining your health records before asking for or attending any meeting at the hospital.

- The General Data Protection Regulation (GDPR) is an EU law on data protection and privacy for all individuals within the European Union.[2] The new framework in place from May 2018 replaced the previous 1995 data protection directive. Note that this law only relates to personal data of a living individual, so rules for obtaining records of those deceased might incur costs.

- If there has been a maternal death, the hospital concerned should carry out a serious incident review or confidential enquiry. There is some criticism of these in a systematic review[3] and it appears that family is not often involved (only 14%). In 60% of cases there was a documented review, in a further 16% the review was mentioned in case notes but was not available, and in 24% there was no review mentioned. The hospital must provide information to the confidential enquiry which reviews all maternal deaths which take place in the UK and Ireland[4].

- If you are concerned about the hospital's or GP surgery's practices regarding management of your personal data, you can report it to the Information Commissioner's Office (ICO). For example, if you have had a problem accessing your information or it is wrong, or they have lost it or disclosed it to someone else – you can report it. Their website[5] has a live chat opportunity or a helpline 0303 1213 1113.

---

2 During the 11-month transition period to 31st December 2020, GDPR will continue to apply in the UK.

3 *BMJ Open* Jun 2019, 9 (6) e029552; DOI: 10.1136/bmjopen-2019-029552

4 National Perinatal Epidemiology Unit (NPEU) MBRRACE reports, *www.npeu. ox.ac.uk/mbrrace-uk*

5 Information Commissioner's Office (ICO), *https://ico.org.uk*

- You may find it interesting and informative to make a Freedom of Information request (FOI) for hospital policies, guidelines and statistics. The following website, *www.gov.uk/make-a-freedom-of-information-request* gives you more information. You can specify that you do not wish your personal details to be passed to other departments and that you would like to be contacted by email only so you do not receive unexpected phone calls from hospital staff.

Once you have received a copy of your health records

Having a copy of the notes at home means that you can go through them at your own pace. If reading the notes makes you feel anxious, angry or uneasy, you can put them away and revisit them at a time that suits you, and/or you can seek help. Some people find it helpful to go through the maternity notes with a doula or an independent midwife, usually for a small fee. This is a gentle way to go through the details at your own pace and get more insight into what should or shouldn't have happened. Or you can use the Patient Advice and Liaison Service (PALS) who are available at your local hospital.

When you have studied your notes, you may find that the staff had good reasons for their actions. Equally you may find issues that you should complain about. For example, there may be entries which are untrue or inaccurate, or entries made by staff who were not present.

If you want an investigation into what happened and you find that the notes are factually incorrect you have the right to have the notes corrected, or a note from you inserted with your view of the events. You can arrange to view the originals at the hospital, especially if you decide to make a complaint. You can do this before receiving the copies, but you can also ask to see them afterwards.

If you are concerned that you may not be able to understand the terminology or jargon of the health records you could

» Look it up online – terminology is exceptionally well-explained on the *Which? Birth Choice* website by well-respected experts in maternity services. See *www.which.co.uk/birth-choice*.

» Ask the NHS Complaints Advocacy Service *https://nhscomplaintsadvocacy.or*g.

» Ask your local Patient Advice and Liaison Service (PALS).

» Ask a local antenatal teacher, maybe through the National Childbirth Trust (NCT).

Please note that a debrief at the hospital is not recommended if you are experiencing anxiety or Post Traumatic Stress Disorder (PTSD) symptoms. Revisiting the original place and event of trauma in a non-therapeutic setting may trigger or worsen PTSD symptoms. (*See Chapter 5, Understanding Birth Trauma.*)

Always be kind to yourself and have some self-care routines and supportive people in place when revisiting events of the birth. It is normal to experience strong emotions, so give yourself time and space to process the information.

Chapter 11

Making a formal complaint

It is a pledge from the **NHS Constitution that

> "When mistakes happen or if you are harmed while receiving health care you receive an appropriate explanation and apology, delivered with sensitivity and recognition of the trauma you have experienced, and know that lessons will be learned to help avoid a similar incident occurring again."

The duty of candour is a statutory duty applying to any organisation carrying out health and/or social care activities which are regulated by the Care Quality Commission, and if a patient is harmed when receiving health care that they will be given a full explanation and offered an apology. This explanation and apology should be given with sensitivity recognising any trauma that the patient may have suffered. There should be an acknowledgment that lessons will be learned to help avoid a similar incident occurring again.

There are four health services in the United Kingdom; NHS England, NHS Scotland, HSC Northern Ireland and NHS Wales. For a good description of how each organisation, together with the NMC and GMC, has considered the duty of candour see *www.nmc.org.uk/standards/guidance/ the-professional-duty-of-candour/read-the-professional-duty-of-candour/*.

**NHS Constitution for England, updated 14th October 2015, *www.gov.uk/government/publications/the-nhs-constitution-for-england/the-nhs-constitution-for-england*

Time limits for negative feedback

Complaints should normally be made within 12 months of an incident or of the matter coming to your attention. It is, however, not uncommon for people to be so traumatised that they cannot face addressing their experiences for many months (and in some cases many years). If you are considering making a complaint but feel unable to within the 12 month period, it is a good idea to send the Patient Advice and Liaison Service (PALS) of the Trust an email "I intend making a complaint about the care I experienced but I am not well enough to deal with it at the moment. I shall take action as soon as I feel able". Wherever possible, do not send this statement before you have obtained a copy of your health records (*see Chapter 10*). The letter will ensure that you are within the deadline and the Trust will be obliged to investigate under the complaints procedures.

This time limit should not, however, inhibit you from writing your complaint even if a year or so has passed; when you have valid reasons for not complaining within the deadline and your complaint is a serious one, this limit should be extended. AIMS recommends that you always make your complaint in writing and keep a copy of the letter.

Complaints need to be sent to different organisations depending on which of the four countries in the UK you live in. The names and addresses of the relevant organisations are listed in Appendix 1 at the back of this book. The addresses are up-to-date at the time of publication but please let us know if you find they have changed.

How to write a formal complaint

First, obtain a copy of the Complaints Procedure at your local hospital or GP practice. This should also be available online. It may say that you should write to the Patient Services Team or similar name. If you have to complete a form, print it off and attach it to your letter (later in this chapter). Although AIMS recommends writing directly to the Chief Executive Officer of the hospital or Trust, you may find that bureaucracy dictates that you must write to the Patient Services team first to get the complaint lodged but there is no harm in copying in the Chief Executive!

If you have been able to write your own account of what happened during your maternity care, (as suggested in previous chapters), this may help you prepare a letter of complaint in which you identify the key issues that you want addressed. If possible, your letter should not exceed three sides of A4 paper. If there are important and specific questions you want answered, make sure they are clearly numbered. If the response to your letter fails to address any of them, it is easier in your next letter to say, "Thank you for the information, however, you have not answered questions 5, 6 and 7". Make your complaint as detailed but as succinct as possible, and include the names of those staff involved or describe them if you don't know their names. Try to write dispassionately – as if you were writing about someone else. It is perfectly acceptable to explain how the incident has affected you, your baby, your relationships, your family and your work.

Your letter can hold the recipient to account by pointing out that not only has something gone wrong, but also by highlighting **where their own standards have not been met**. The complaint should contain the following:-

- Your name and address, and if you don't mind being contacted by phone or email, give those too. If you do mind, state clearly that you wish to be contacted via written correspondence only and do not include a telephone number. Requesting written correspondence only will give you the most control as you have time to consider the responses and there is no ambiguity as to what has been discussed.

- Your hospital and NHS numbers.
- A factual account of what happened, including the time and place where any evidence you may have occurred.
- Details of who was involved. These should be in your notes, but if you do not have the names of the people involved, try to describe their physical appearance or give the date and time that they were on duty. Describe their behaviour, but do not make any personal comments about them.
- How it has affected you or your baby.
  - ○ Give as many details as possible, including mental and physical harm.
- Ask the specific questions for which you need answers.

Be very clear as to what you would like to happen as a result of your complaint. For example, would you like

- a full investigation and for you to be informed of the outcome
- an apology in writing or in person
- an acknowledgement that something went wrong
- an explanation in writing or in a meeting.

You might want someone to be disciplined or prosecuted, but this is not usually possible. If your complaint is upheld, the person may be disciplined but you may not be told (for reasons of staff confidentiality). If you believe the person guilty of professional misconduct or physical assault, you have the option to report them to their professional body and the police (*see Chapter 12, Not satisfied? Where next?*).

Then finish by saying:

- I expect an acknowledgement of receipt of my complaint within 3 working days please with an indication of the period within which the investigation is likely to be completed and a response sent, and to have it properly investigated under your duty of candour.

We suggest you are succinct and factual without sounding emotional. This is because the person reading it, at this stage, needs to understand quickly how important, serious and urgent your complaint is, rather than how you feel about it.

At AIMS we believe that complaints will be more powerful if you can link them to the standards and requirements that midwives and doctors are supposed to follow. The following examples show you how to make your letter more effective.

» Use the Human Rights Act 1998

You should be able to find a relevant quote (*see Chapter 1*) for your situation. For example:

"I believe you have shown a lack of respect for my dignity whilst I was giving birth – this is contrary to Article 8 of the Human Rights Act 1998."

See *www.birthrights.org.uk/library/factsheets/Human-Rights-in-Maternity-Care.pdf*

» Informed consent is a legal requirement

"Staff named … did not seek my consent to …"

See *www.birthrights.org.uk/factsheets/consenting-to-treatment/*

» It is a woman's legal right to choose where to give birth

"You denied me my choice of where to give birth … "

See *www.birthrights.org.uk/factsheets/choice-of-place-of-birth/*

» Challenge by quoting Professional Standards

You may find a relevant quote for your situation from **the NMC code of conduct for midwives.** For example:

I understand from the NMC Code of Practice[1] Para 2.5 and 2.6 that the midwife named ... should have respected, supported and documented my right to refuse the care and treatment offered to me, and moreover that she could see I was in distress and so should have responded compassionately and politely, rather than ..."

The GMC code of conduct for doctors is called Good Medical Practice[2]:

I understand from the Good Medical Practice Code (the link above will take you to the code) Para 31, that the female doctor named ... should have listened to me, taken account of my views and responded honestly to my questions instead of telling me to leave it to her to decide, because she knew best. Therefore she is required to put matters right/offer an apology/explain what happened, fully and promptly, and justify why she spoke to me in that way.

» Use information from the Better Births Report[3]

I note from the report Better Births: Improving outcomes of maternity services in England A Five Year Forward View for maternity care (February 2016):

"Our vision for maternity services across England is for them to become safer, more personalised, kinder, professional and more family friendly; where every woman has access to information to enable her to make decisions about her care; and where she and her baby can access support that is centred around their individual needs and circumstances. And for all staff to be supported to deliver care which is women-centred, working in high performing teams,

1 *www.nmc.org.uk/standards/code/read-the-code-online*

2 *www.gmc-uk.org/ethical-guidance/ethical-guidance-for-doctors/good-medical-practice*

3 *www.england.nhs.uk/wp-content/uploads/2017/12/implementing-better-births.pdf*

in organisations which are well led and in cultures which promote innovation, continuous learning, and break down organisational and professional boundaries."

I hope you will bear this in mind when reviewing my complaint.

Other information you could use from this report:

I was given an episiotomy – the Implementing Better Births report (2018) clearly states that if I had had continuity of carer I would have been 16% less likely to have needed one.

I believe my care was compromised as there was no one midwife responsible for liaising with my cardiologist, as suggested in the Implementing Better Births report (2018). This resulted in ...

I had treatment from x (give a number) different midwives during my pregnancy – the Implementing Better Births report (2018) recommends that "an on-going relationship built on trust gives the woman more confidence to be open with her midwife...". I believe that I would have been less likely to (briefly summarise what your complaint is about) had I had the same named midwife to care for me throughout my pregnancy, birth and postnatal period.

It may be a good idea to get help with writing and proofreading your letter to make sure everything is clear – perhaps ask a member of your family or a friend, or Citizens Advice which have offices in most towns.

An example of a letter to send

Your home address

*Email address

*If you do not mind being contacted by email,
give your email address as well.

Name and address of the person
you are writing to   Date

Dear

Your Name, Date of Birth and Hospital Number

I am writing to make a formal complaint about the treatment I
received in **WARD, HOSPITAL** on **DATE** and I am holding you
accountable to investigate and to report back to me in a timely
manner.

*Make the bullet points below into paragraphs and give DETAILS of what happened
to you.*

- The main events in date and time order.
- The staff involved – names or descriptions.
- A brief description of how it has affected you and/or your
  baby, including any mental or physical harm – if you have
  several items, list the most important first. Be clear and
  concise.
- Any evidence you may have (perhaps from your case notes)
  and from any witnesses, for example your partner, doula or
  independent midwife.

*State HOW the staff/hospital may have BROKEN THEIR OWN RULES or
GUIDELINES, if you think they did. This is where you might use the phrases and
references listed in the previous section.*

For example:

I believe [staff names]...... have shown a lack of respect for my
dignity whilst I was giving birth, in violation of Article 8 of the
Human Rights Act 1998.

ASK THE QUESTIONS you would like answered, and number them.
For example:

1. Why did Midwife [name] carry on giving me a vaginal examination when I had not given my consent?
2. Why did the Obstetrician [name] insist that I was induced by telling me my baby might die if I refused?
3. Why was my partner told to leave the room?

DETAILS OF WHAT YOU WOULD LIKE TO HAPPEN as a result of your complaint. For example:

I would like Dr [name] to apologise to me face to face **OR** give me a written apology, and explain to me why the following procedure [xxxxxx] to which I did not consent was carried out **AND** provide evidence for the need for [xxxxxx] in my circumstance.

I expect an acknowledgement of receipt of my complaint within 3 working days please, with an indication of the period within which the investigation is likely to be completed and a response sent, and to have it properly investigated as is my right under your duty of candour.

Yours sincerely,

Signature and date
Print your full name

Ask someone to proofread your letter, keep copies of it and send one by 'Signed For: Proof of Delivery' at the Post Office; you will then have confirmation that it has been received.

What happens next

You should receive an acknowledgement within 2-3 working days confirming that your complaint has been received and indicating what should happen next. You should normally receive a response to your complaint within 6 months, and be informed of its progress. The response should include how the complaint was dealt with, whether there was an investigation, what the conclusions were and what if any action is to be taken. If they accept that mistakes have been made you should receive an apology. Be aware that you cannot be offered any compensation, you must take legal action to receive compensation. (*See Chapter 13 Legal Action for Maternity Cases.*)

An offer to meet with the staff

The response to the complaint may include an offer to meet with the staff to try to resolve your complaint. AIMS recommends that you prepare carefully for this meeting and take someone with you.

You do not have to have a face-to-face meeting with the staff involved if you do not wish to; equally you may request a meeting if you feel it would help to resolve your complaint. Sometimes parents attend the meeting expecting to meet the staff directly involved only to find that another consultant or manager is there in their place. You should ask ahead of the meeting who will be there. Complaints can cover obstetric, midwifery or paediatric care and it would be preferable for a representative from each specialism involved to be there i.e. the consultant obstetrician, the Director of Midwifery, the consultant paediatrician, as well as an administrator, whichever is appropriate.

You can agree to attend the meeting, but establish in advance that the minutes of the meeting will be taken, that you will receive a copy and that a letter will be written to you responding to the points you raised. These meetings can be very stressful; take a recording device and ask if you can record the meeting because you are likely to forget all that is said. Anecdotally, AIMS has been told by women that taking in recording devices appears to make the meetings less confrontational.

Chapter 12

Not satisfied? Where next?

If you are not satisfied with the outcome of your complaint to the hospital trust, there are people and organisations that you can contact.

To complain about a midwife or nurse's professional practice or conduct

If your complaint is about a specific member of staff whom you believe has been unprofessional or incompetent you may wish to complain directly to their professional bodies. This is the NMC for nurses and midwives.

Nursing and Midwifery Council (NMC)

Midwives are registered with this professional regulatory body *www.nmc.org.uk*. The website advises that it is best to raise your concerns with the employer (the hospital trust where the midwife works) first. However, if you have concerns about reporting to the employer for any reason and you believe that the midwife potentially poses a threat to patient safety, matters should be reported directly to NMC. Raise your concerns as soon as possible, but there are no time limits. In serious cases, it may be necessary to act quickly to stop the midwife from working or restrict their practice until the case is investigated. If the midwife is a serious risk to the public or themselves, you can make a referral to the NMC AND the employer immediately. The NMC investigate allegations including:

- misconduct
- lack of competence
- criminal behaviour
- not having the necessary knowledge of English
- serious ill health.

The NMC's Code of Practice sets out the professional standards that midwives must uphold in order to be registered to practice in the UK. Being 'fit to practice' requires a midwife to have the skills, knowledge, health and character to do their job safely and effectively. If an allegation is made that the standards required were not met, the midwife will be investigated and, if proven to be true, may be sanctioned or removed from the register (known as 'struck off').

There is a Public referral form to complete online. It will be received by the screening team and you will be given details of what happens next. There is detailed information on the NMC website (*www.nmc.org.uk*).

In 2018, the NMC launched a new service called the Public Support Service so if you raise a complaint about a midwife you should receive one-to-one support from the beginning from a dedicated, named individual who will guide you through the process. The NMC are committed

> " ... to listening to people's concerns and giving them a voice when things go wrong with their care, treating them with the respect, compassion and the humanity they deserve."[1]

---

1 Jessie Cunnett, Head of Public Support Service, NMC. Press release, 8 December 2018 *www.nmc.org.uk/news/press-releases/nmc-launches-new-support-service/*

To complain about a doctor's professional practice or conduct

Contact the General Medical Council (GMC)

All doctors are registered with this Council, *www.gmc-uk.org*, including all grades of doctors e.g. consultants, registrars and all junior staff, and all disciplines, e.g. obstetricians, paediatricians and general practitioners (GPs).

The website has clear guidance on how the Council handles concerns from the public. Please note: the GMC website uses the term 'concern' to cover very serious offences. If you raise a complaint with them they are very likely to refer to the employer to establish what has happened. They state that their focus is on the most serious complaints that could put patients at risk or lose the public's confidence in the medical profession.

The GMC investigate allegations including:

- serious or repeated mistakes in patient care
- failure to respond reasonably to patient needs (e.g. not referring for further investigations where necessary)
- violence, sexual assault or indecency
- fraud or dishonesty
- a serious criminal offence
- abuse of professional position (e.g. an improper sexual relationship with a patient)
- discrimination against patients, colleagues and others
- serious breaches of patient confidentiality
- serious concerns about knowledge of English.

There is an online referral form to make a complaint about a doctor or to complain on someone else's behalf. The advice on the GMC website includes what to expect and what the outcome may be.

Who oversees the NMC and GMC?

Professional Standards Authority (PSA)

The **PSA** has the responsibility to oversee the regulators' Councils, e.g. the NMC and GMC, and is able to review the decisions made by all the nine regulators about practitioners' fitness to practice. You can visit their website *www.professionalstandards.org.uk* to check the names and registration of any doctor or midwife or other health professional. Every professional working in or out of the Health Service is required to have up-to-date registration.

The PSA would like to hear about your experiences with a regulator, in particular where you have contacted them about the 'fitness to practice' of an individual. Go to *www.professionalstandards.org.uk/share-your-experience/share-your-experience-of-regulators*.

The PSA also set the standards or guidance for people working in the health sector so it is worth reading their website as it may be worth quoting from their standards in your complaint. However, the PSA may review correspondence between the NMC or GMC and the public, but they cannot intervene on specific cases.

Were you affected by a commissioning decision?

Clinical Commissioning Group (CCG)

CCGs are clinically-led statutory NHS organisations responsible for the planning, commissioning and monitoring of health care services in a local area. This means that they must plan for all the maternity services in their area – including how many midwives and obstetricians are needed, care for vulnerable women, antenatal and postnatal mental health and breastfeeding (this is only a fraction of all the things they need to think about).

The NCT/RCM/RCOG have an easy to read guide to *Making Sense of Commissioning Maternity Services in England*[2].

They must commission maternity services with the local Trust or Trusts and then monitor how those Trusts achieve the requirements of the contract.

If you have a complaint or concern relating to the way an NHS service has been commissioned or you have been directly affected by a commissioning decision (this may include local hospital policies or funding decisions, for example) you can contact the complaints team in your local CCG. The CGC will explain whether they think they are well-placed to deal with your complaint and give you the information on how to complain. The procedure should be very similar to that at the hospital (*see page 109*).

Reporting your concerns about the maternity service?

Care Quality Commission (CQC)

The CQC have a new campaign called #DeclareYourCare (join the conversation on Instagram and Twitter). "After new research found that almost 7 million people who have used health or social care services in the last five years have had concerns about their care but never raised them. Of these, over half (58%) expressed regret about not doing so."

The CQC has set up an on-line referral form to make it easy to report your concern (you can report good care too) as well as make a complaint to the provider of your care. The CQC says it will use the information practically because it helps them to decide what, when and where to inspect, perhaps making it urgent to do so. However, they cannot support you to make a complaint or take it up on your behalf.

---

2 *www.nct.org.uk/sites/default/files/related_documents/Advice%20to%20CCGs%20final%20version.pdf*

The CQC will let you know that they have received your information and may get in touch with you for further details. You will not be told what happens on an individual basis, but you can sign up for email alerts which will tell you if an inspection report has been made on a particular local care service. Sign up at *www.cqc.org.uk/news/newsletters-alerts/our-email-alerts* #DeclareYourCare at *www.cqc.org.uk/get-involved/share-your-experience/peoples-experience-care-what-we-want-know-why*.

Were you discriminated against?

The Equality and Human Rights Commission

The Commission is responsible for monitoring and enforcing the Public Sector Equality Duty (*see Chapter 4, Putting your experience into context*). If you feel that you have been discriminated against and it falls within the jurisdiction of this Commission, then you can apply for a judicial review in relation to a breach of this duty. More guidance can be found at *www.equalityhumanrights.com* and you can speak or write to the Equality Advisory and Support Service at *www.equalityadvisoryservice.com*.

Are you dissatisfied with the response to your complaint to the hospital trust?

Complain to the ombudsman responsible for health

www.ombudsman.org.uk/

If you are dissatisfied with the response to your complaint you can appeal to the relevant ombudsman for England, Wales, Northern Ireland or Scotland – see Appendix 1. There is a time limit of one year from when you "became aware of the problem", so do not delay sending your appeal. They can extend the deadline if, for example, the complaint took much longer than usual to investigate, or your health prevented you from complaining earlier. If you are finding it too difficult to address your issues you can write to the ombudsman and inform them that you intend to lodge a complaint but that you are not able to submit details at this time and you will do so as soon as you feel able.

The ombudsman is able to determine the care they would expect, according to relevant guidelines and standards, the care you experienced (with reference to your health records and explanations from both you and the organisation), whether there is a difference between the two that constitutes a failing, and what more, if anything, may be needed to put this right.

The ombudsman will need to know if you are intending to take legal action, because the law says that they cannot investigate a complaint if you have (or had) the option to do this. But the law also says they can be flexible so they will look at your individual circumstances. The ombudsman can investigate if the subject of the legal action is different to that which you want them to investigate. e.g. your complaint to the ombudsman may be about the way the Trust dealt with your complaint or about the attitudes of the midwife involved with your care, but your legal action is about the negligence of a doctor.

The Parliamentary and Health Service ombudsman for England has a document called the ombudsman Casework Assurance Process[3] which clearly states that if "a complaint about a service or decision from an MP (or MP supported), or if an MP has a specific interest in the case or asks the ombudsman to take interest" then that complaint meets the criteria for "potential specific handling or oversight" – in other words, goes straight to the top of the pile! There are other criteria too in that document which you might like to read. They also have a process to deal with Tweets on the ombudsman or CEO's Twitter account!

---

3 *www.ombudsman.org.uk/sites/default/files/page/Ombudsman%20Casework%20 Assurance%20process_0.pdf*

Talk to your MP

It is really worthwhile meeting with your MP in their 'surgery' to tell them that you have complained and what the response has been. They should be able to help you by writing to the hospital or indeed, the ombudsman, which may in turn bring your complaint to the top of the pile. Hopefully, by informing your MP, they may be able to recognise a rising trend in complaints/concerns raised by local patients. (*See also 'Complain to the ombudsman for health', p76.*)

Take legal action

See Chapter 13 for a brief overview of the implications of bringing a court case.

Problem accessing your health records?

Information Commissioner

If you have had a problem accessing your health records, or have a concern about the way it has been held, its accuracy or its security, you can report it ("within three months of your last meaningful contact with the organisation concerned") to the Information Commissioner. Use the website *https://ico.org.uk/make-a-complaint/your-personal-information-concerns/* to complete the details of your concern.

An issue of patient safety?

Reporting Assault to the Police

If you have experienced a violation of informed consent such as an unconsented-to vaginal examination, or if you were held down or hit by staff, you may wish to report the assault to the police. Carrying out a procedure without consent is assault, which could potentially be a crime or 'civil wrong'. However, and this is important, if there is no physical injury sustained (and this probably needs to be quite severe) it may be harder for the police to pursue a case. Criminal law does not appear to be as concerned with mental injury. In civil law there is not yet case law for mental injury sustained as a result of lack of care in pregnancy or birth, so solicitors may not take cases on.

As you may imagine this is a very difficult area of law to explain - medical and clinical procedures have outcomes which are often devastating but without meeting definitions for 'medical or clinical negligence' or 'sexual offences', it is unlikely the police will be able to pursue a case. The law needs to change to recognise that such a thing as 'obstetric violence' does exist in reality.

You can make an appointment to see the Chief Inspector by phoning the police station so it will be at a time and date that suits you. Always go with someone that can offer you support. Take a written statement about what happened and witness statements if you have any as this will be helpful. It is also helpful to have your maternity notes with you in case further details are required. Ask for a police reference number and the name of the person you talked to.

You can report the incident regardless of whether you would like to press charges. Reporting incidents to the police is an important step in recognising "obstetric violence". It took a long time for domestic violence to be recognised as a criminal offence. Raising awareness and reporting harms caused by violent behaviour of medical staff is an important first step into changing the culture and hopefully, one day, changing the law.

A serious untoward incident

NHS Trusts are required to report all serious incidents to whoever is responsible for commissioning maternity services in your area (this will usually be the local CCG in England). Such incidents are categorised as "any unintended or unexpected incident which could have or did lead to harm for one or more patients receiving NHS care".

There is national guidance[4] about the reporting process. If you have a complaint which you think amounts to a serious incident you can write to the Trust and ask them for a copy of their policy on serious incidents and ask them to provide evidence that they have done what they were supposed to do.

NHS Improvement

This department collects and analyses information on patient safety incidents in the NHS in England. They then make recommendations to reduce the risk of patient safety incidents. They do not investigate each report individually but they provide feedback to the health service as a whole from time to time, based on their analysis and findings from all reports as a whole. If you are not satisfied with the response you have had from the Trust then you may wish to consider alerting NHS Improvement and asking them to investigate. They can be contacted via their website (*https://improvement.nhs.uk/contact-us/*) or you can write to them directly or telephone their Helpline on 0300 123 2257 and inform them that you are a patient who wishes to report a serious incident.

The equivalent body in Northern Ireland is called the Northern Ireland Adverse Incident Centre[5], in Scotland is known as Healthcare Improvement Scotland[6] and in Wales, the relevant body is Patient Safety Wales[7].

---

4 *https://improvement.nhs.uk/resources/serious-incident-framework/*

5 *www.health-ni.gov.uk/topics/safety-and-quality-standards/northern-ireland-adverse-incident-centre-niaic*

6 *www.healthcareimprovementscotland.org/about_us/contact_us.aspx*

7 *www.patientsafety.wales.nhs.uk/about-us*

A death has occurred

Coroner

A death in hospital should be reported if "there is a question of negligence or misadventure about the treatment of the person who died".

Coroners are independent judicial officers who investigate deaths reported to them. They will make the inquiries necessary to establish the cause of death, this includes ordering a post-mortem examination, obtaining witness statements and medical records, or holding an inquest. (For more information about when a baby dies, see Chapter 7, Why did my baby die?)

Final resort?

Clinical Ethics Committees

Your local hospital trust may have a Clinical Ethics Committee (as opposed to a Research Ethics Committee which is set up to agree and monitor research proposals), whose function is policy development, education and consultation, see *www.ukcen.net/main/about*. AIMS has no experience of using these committees to discuss ethical issues in pregnancy and childbirth but it is possible that you have a case which is appropriate for referral to your local committee. You may even be invited to participate in the discussion. However, Sheila A M McLean warns in her article 'What and who are clinical ethics committees for?'[8] that there may be a conflict of interest for the committee which is primarily set up as a multi-disciplinary forum for discussion of issues, supporting the decision-making of health professionals.

Basically, however strange it may seem, the interests or focus of health professionals and patients may not be the same. There should be a lay member

---

8 'What and who are clinical ethics committees for?', Sheila A M McLean, *Journal of Medical Ethics*, (2000) Sep; 33(9): 497-500 *www.ncbi.nlm.nih.gov/pmc/articles/PMC2080817/*

on the committee and AIMS recommends contacting that person for advice. These committees are strictly advisory, but it is said that families and staff benefit from the service, *www.bmj.com/content/328/7445/950/rapid-responses.*

However, because these committees are advisory they will vary in quality substantially, and are not bound by any constraints. Note that it is not a requirement for all hospitals to have a clinical ethics committee and even if they do, they may not take up a case referred by a patient or even ask a patient to be present in a discussion. On the other hand you might be lucky and find an enlightened committee willing to discuss the ethical issue you may have.

Chapter 13

Legal action for maternity cases

Legal reparation is, no doubt, a difficult route to go down for seeking resolution for a wrongful act. But justice may be achieved by using the laws regarding clinical negligence and the Human Rights Act. I have invited two guest authors to explain briefly about the laws and how they can work for you. I am delighted that Liz Thomas, Policy and Research Manager from AvMA (Action against Medical Accidents) and Elizabeth Prochaska, Chair of Trustees at Birthrights have agreed to write for us in this chapter.

Embarking on any kind of legal case can be a very daunting prospect and it is particularly so if you are also coping with the emotional and physical consequences of negligent care. The first step is to get the right advice and support to help you decide what course of action would be best for you and your family. Pursuing a legal claim is not the right option for everyone but an experienced solicitor should be able to help you make a decision and to guide you through the process.

AvMA is a charity which "... supports people affected by avoidable harm in health care; to help them achieve justice; and to promote better patient safety for all". It provides a free advice and information service with a team of trained volunteers working through AvMA's helpline and a small team of in-house advisors with medical or legal backgrounds who advise on more complex written casework and inquests. Their website is *www.avma.org.uk*.

Birthrights provides advice and information to women about their maternity care, campaigns to change maternity policy and systems and provides practical training on rights-respecting care to doctors and midwives. They have an understanding of the legal issues in maternity care and insight into the emotional needs of women at this time. Their website is *www.birthrights.org.uk*.

Liz Thomas, Policy and Research Manager from AvMA writes...

The birth of a new baby is normally a time of joy and celebration for the parents and the extended family but in a very small number of cases, the outcome is not as expected because either the mother or baby experiences harm. This could be the result of an unavoidable complication of pregnancy or childbirth and is no one's fault. However, there will be some instances where the mother or baby suffers an avoidable injury as a result of failures in the care provided during pregnancy, labour or in the neonatal period. When this happens, it can be a very difficult and overwhelming time. You may be worrying about the future and how you will cope both practically and financially with the consequences of what has happened. As a result, in addition to wanting to find out what went wrong and why, one option you may also be considering is whether you can obtain compensation.

There is no automatic entitlement to compensation. You would in most instances need to instruct a lawyer to investigate and pursue a legal claim for clinical negligence against the healthcare provider. This is not a decision to be taken lightly as it can be a long and sometimes difficult process but it may also be seen as a necessity, for example, to secure funding to meet your child's future care needs or to compensate you for the financial consequences of what has happened if you are unable to work due to a significant physical or psychological injury.

How can I find out what happened and if I might have a claim?

If you or your baby have suffered harm, a number of different investigations may be taking place which may help to provide an explanation of what happened and why. The type of investigation and who carries it out will in part depend on the nature and seriousness of the harm that has been caused as well as where your care was provided. For example, private maternity care is dealt with differently to NHS care and different arrangements apply across the four nations of the United Kingdom.

Most maternity incidents will be investigated by the healthcare provider themselves. This could be in response to a complaint you have made or an internal investigation initiated by the healthcare provider. There is also a duty of candour requiring healthcare professionals (UK wide) and healthcare organisations (in England and Scotland) to be open and honest with patients and notify them if it is believed avoidable harm may have been caused.

In addition to any investigations being carried out by the healthcare provider itself, some NHS maternity cases in England may also be subject to external investigations by the Healthcare Safety Investigation Branch (HSIB) as well as by NHS Resolution.

HSIB is tasked with undertaking detailed maternity investigations in relation to cases where a mother has died during pregnancy or shortly thereafter; in cases where the baby has suffered a significant brain injury; or where the baby has died during or after labour. HSIB will seek the consent of the family to undertake an investigation and the family can choose how involved they want to be in the process. If the family does not give their consent, the investigation will revert to the NHS Trust involved. At the end of the HSIB investigation, the family will receive a report setting out the findings of the investigation. (*See website www.hsib.org.*)

If there is evidence to suggest that a baby may have suffered a potentially serious brain injury at or around the time of birth and the care was provided by the NHS in England, the healthcare provider is required to report the case to NHS Resolution under their Early Notification Scheme (ENS). NHS Resolution is the body responsible for managing and defending legal claims against the NHS in England. The investigation by NHS Resolution could in some cases result in an early admission of fault (liability) and enable you to obtain compensation for your baby without having to first prove negligence. If your baby's case is being investigated under the Early Notification Scheme, you would still be strongly advised to get independent legal advice on behalf of your baby from a solicitor experienced in birth injury cases. They can advise you on the findings of the investigation including if further investigations would be warranted as well as advising you on the compensation your child would be entitled to.

Where a mother or baby has died and there is evidence to suggest the death may have been avoidable, the case should be reported to the local coroner. It is also open to the family to raise any concerns they have directly with the coroner. The coroner may hold an inquest (a public hearing) to examine the circumstances and to determine the cause of death. In Scotland, the Procurator Fiscal is responsible for investigating deaths by holding a Fatal Accident Inquiry.

The outcome of these investigations as well as any complaint you make to the hospital or healthcare provider should help provide you with that all–important explanation of what happened and why. If you are thinking about legal action, it may also help you and your solicitor identify whether there are grounds to pursue a legal claim. If you contact AvMA, their advisors can give you advice about all these various processes.

How do I find the right solicitor for my case?

Clinical negligence is a specialist area of law where the experience and expertise of your lawyer can make a significant difference to the outcome of your case. Both AvMA and the Law Society have accredited specialist clinical negligence lawyers but you should also ask the lawyer about their experience of successfully conducting cases similar to yours. For example, if the case involves a baby that has died, it can make the legal process a little easier if you have a solicitor who understands and is sensitive to the needs of bereaved parents.

How will my case be investigated?

For a legal claim to be successful, it is necessary to prove not only that the care provided was below an acceptable standard, but that the failures in care were directly responsible for the injuries for which compensation is being claimed. The main evidence in support of a claim will come from medical experts instructed by your solicitor. These will be senior doctors, midwives and other relevant healthcare professionals who will usually be experienced in providing opinions in clinical negligence claims. A claim will only proceed and have any chance of success if it has the support of your medical experts.

How long will a legal claim take?

If the healthcare provider accepts responsibility (liability) for your claim, it may be possible to settle your claim at a relatively early stage but this could still take at least two to three years. If the case involves a child, it may be necessary to keep the claim open for a number of years in order to determine what the child's needs might be in the future. If the healthcare provider denies you have a valid claim but your solicitor and barrister advising on your case believes the claim has good prospects of success, the solicitor will need to issue legal proceedings within the legal time limit and it could then take several more years before the outcome of the claim is known.

What is the time limit for pursuing a clinical negligence claim?

There is a 3-year time limit for issuing a claim for clinical negligence which runs from the date of the alleged negligence. If you were unaware at the time that you had been harmed, the three years runs from the date when you first realised you had suffered an injury. However, you should always confirm this with a solicitor as early as possible, particularly if you think you may already be outside the legal time limit. Although the time limit is three years, you should always aim to instruct a solicitor at least one to two years before the time limit expires to allow time for the claim to be investigated. In the case of harm to children, the 3-year time limit does not start to run until the child is 18 years of age (age 16 in Scotland) but you would normally want to start a claim on their behalf as early as possible whilst memories of what happened are still fresh. It also means that if the claim is successful, you can get financial help with meeting your child's care needs whilst they are still young.

If the claim involves someone who due to mental incapacity was unable to manage their own affairs prior to or as a result of the alleged negligence, the 3-year period doesn't apply until (and unless) they regain capacity but again this should be confirmed by a specialist solicitor as the law around legal time limits (limitation) can be complex. In very rare cases, the courts do have powers to allow a claim to proceed outside these time limits but this is not frequently exercised and so should not be relied on.

How will the legal costs be paid?

There are a number of options for paying the costs of investigating a clinical negligence claim. In England and Wales, most clinical negligence cases are funded by conditional fee agreements (CFAs or 'no win, no fee agreements') but some cases may be funded through legal expenses insurance which is included in some household insurance policies. Legal aid is available but only for claims on behalf of children who have suffered a significant neurological injury at or around the time of birth. This would include brain injuries as well as other significant neurological injuries such as Erb's Palsy but not other types of injury to the baby. Different funding arrangements apply in Scotland and Northern Ireland. You can find details of the various options for funding legal action on AvMA's website as well as on individual law firms' websites. If your claim is successful, most of the legal costs will be paid by the healthcare provider but particularly in relation to CFAs, you will usually have to pay a proportion of the costs out of your compensation. It is important that the solicitor explains all of this at the outset of your case.

Wrongful birth claims

There is an additional group of birth-related cases referred to as wrongful birth claims. These claims arise where negligent care before or during pregnancy has resulted in the birth of a child who would not otherwise have been born. This could be due to a negligently performed sterilisation, vasectomy or termination of pregnancy where you can claim for the costs of an unwanted pregnancy. A wrongful birth claim can also arise where there has been a failure to diagnose and warn the parents about a serious congenital defect where the parents would have otherwise chosen to terminate the pregnancy. The claim would be for the additional costs of bringing up a child with a disability. The 3-year time limit applies to wrongful birth claims as it is the parents' claim and not the child's.

Elizabeth Prochaska, Chair of Birthrights explains…

Human rights claims

If you believe that your rights may have been breached during your pregnancy or birth, you may have a claim under the Human Rights Act 1998. The Act prohibits public bodies, including all NHS services, from breaching the rights set out in the European Convention on Human Rights. These include the right not to be subjected to inhuman and degrading treatment, the right to private life, which includes the right to privacy, autonomy and informed consent, and the right to non-discrimination. Here are some examples of breaches of human rights:

- If you were given a vaginal examination without your consent, the doctor or midwife will have violated your right to autonomy and may also have subjected you to inhuman and degrading treatment.

- If your personal details were shared with another person without your consent, or you were physically exposed to others, your right to privacy may have been breached.

- If choices you made about your birth were not respected, the hospital may have breached your right to autonomy and informed consent.

- If you experienced serious neglect on a post-natal ward that led to harm to you or your baby, you might have a claim for inhuman treatment.

If you want to explore making a legal claim for breach of your human rights after your child is born, you will need to contact a solicitor. There is a one year limitation period for these claims and the compensation that can be awarded by the courts is low. For this reason, human rights claims are quite rare and usually brought alongside claims for clinical negligence when there has been harm to the mother or baby.

While human rights claims are not always the most effective way to obtain compensation, human rights can be used to ensure that your choices about birth are respected and you receive the care that you want before your baby is born.

Conclusion

You can see that making a legal claim is not for the fainthearted. However, obtaining your notes and getting as much information as possible from the hospital is a good first step. If staff at the hospital ask if you are likely to take legal action, you could say 'I haven't decided yet'. (If they think you plan to, they may become defensive.) The next step is contacting a solicitor to find out more information. There are people and organisations who will support you. More information about the Human Rights Act and using it to support your complaint is mentioned in 'How to write a formal complaint' in Chapter 11.

Chapter 14

Planning for subsequent births

You may wish to consider the ideas in this chapter for any subsequent birth you are planning, whether you have reached any kind of resolution of your previous birthing experience or not; or you may find yourself with an unplanned pregnancy in which case the steps to consider may be the same or similar. You may be very frightened of the prospect of another birth, and although this is a normal response, you may wish to think about how to cope with the pregnancy and birth.

This information is designed to signpost you to potential sources of support and help for a future birth. Simply reading this chapter is not enough. Women who speak to AIMS tell us that it is crucial to avoid the midwives and doctors and often the institutions that caused the earlier trauma that they are now seeking a resolution to. You should not risk being subjected to further abuse, or having to relive previous experiences. If you cannot think what to do, please email or phone the AIMS helplines.

Most importantly please find some support.

There is no one approach for planning for this pregnancy and birth and there is certainly no consistency from midwives and doctors in dealing with women who have experienced birth trauma. Don't be afraid to decide to birth at home or use a different hospital or birth centre – you have the right to do so. You can insist that you have different midwives and obstetricians from the previous birth. It will be helpful to clearly state this in 'My Birthing Decisions' (see below) saying how important it is to you.

Talk to your consultant obstetrician and midwife

Prepare yourself for this conversation by writing down

- the experiences you had which were key to the trauma you suffered during your last pregnancy or birth
- what you wish to happen this time
- what you need to avoid this time.

If possible, take your partner or someone else with you who knows and understands your history – perhaps another member of your family or a friend or a doula.

The agreements which are made at this meeting must be written down. A summary of what happened to you and your baby in the previous pregnancy and birth should be part of this document so that you do not have to repeat your history every time you see someone new. For the purposes of this book we will call this document 'My Birthing Decisions'. You can write these down yourself and on the next page we give you samples of the different wording and formats depending on what is most important for you.

It is good practice for your consultant and midwife to also give you a written plan which matches your decisions, and will also contain contingency plans if things change. You should remind them that your consent must be obtained if things change. If you have as much information as possible written down, it will, hopefully, give you more control over what may happen.

These two documents should be kept in a prominent place at the front of your maternity notes. Make sure that you and your birth partner(s) have copies too and keep them in your labour bag!

Examples of 'My Birthing Decisions'

These are for you to decide on. You can change your mind before or during labour. If your decision is to have a planned caesarean birth the example about caesarean birth follows this one.

TO WHOM IT MAY CONCERN

As agreed with my Consultant [*name*] and my named Midwife [*name*] on [*date*].

If there is a need to deviate from my decisions during my labour, you must first obtain my consent.

I plan to give birth [*at home, in Birth Centre, in xxxx Ward*], NOT in *xxxxx* where my last baby was born.

You will read in the notes prepared by my consultant and my midwife that my previous birth was traumatic for reasons they explain. That is why I have made these decisions before my labour.

I understand that things may not go as planned, in which case I will wish to speak with my consultant, or another consultant obstetrician who understands my situation, to discuss options.

Thank you for your support.

(*Print your name and sign this statement.*)

(WRITE DOWN YOUR NEEDS and DISCUSS THEM WITH YOUR CONSULTANT AND MIDWIFE. THESE ARE EXAMPLES ONLY.)

My decisions

My birth partner(s) (name/s)

I do not want vaginal examinations at any time

Do not touch me without obtaining my consent

Do not talk to me unless necessary, or I speak to you

Do not offer me pain relief – I will ask for it if I need it

No trainees in the labour room

Keep lights low at all times

During labour

1st stage

I need free movement

I would like to use the birthing pool

I need to shower

I will need food and water

I do not want an IV or cannula

I do not want continuous monitoring

2nd stage

I need free movement and active/upright labour positions

Do not use stirrups

I do not want directed pushing or counting

I do not want an episiotomy

I do not want you to use forceps or vacuum delivery

3rd stage

I want immediate skin-to-skin and support with breastfeeding ASAP

I want delayed cord clamping; birth partner to cut the cord

I want a physiological birth of placenta

My Newborn

Examinations, weighing, cleaning etc., must be when I ask and in my and/or my birth partner's presence

Vitamin K injection – yes/no

I don't want my baby given

Formula

Sugar water

A dummy

~ ~ ~ ~ ~ ~ ~ ~ ~ ~ ~ ~ ~

Examples of 'My Birthing Decisions (planned caesarean)'

TO WHOM IT MAY CONCERN

As agreed with my Consultant [*name*] and my Midwife [*name*] on [*date*].

If there is a need to deviate from my decisions during my labour, you must first obtain my consent. I plan to have a caesarean section on [*date*].

You will read in the notes prepared by my consultant and my midwife that my previous birth was traumatic for reasons they explain. That is why I have made these decisions before birthing.

I understand that things may not go as planned, in which case I will wish speak with my consultant or another consultant obstetrician who understands my situation, to discuss options.

Thank you for your support.

(*Print your name and sign this statement.*)

(THESE ARE EXAMPLES ONLY – WRITE DOWN YOUR NEEDS and DISCUSS THEM WITH YOUR CONSULTANT AND MIDWIFE)

My birth partner(s) names

My decisions

I would like a gentle and natural caesarean.

Please introduce us to the staff who will be caring for me and my baby during the surgery.

I want to be fully aware and conscious, so I request an epidural and no other drugs unless my consent is sought.

Any monitoring of me should be done sensitively.

Please arrange it so that I can see my baby being supported by the doctor to wriggle out of my womb and for my partner and I to see the baby's sex as it emerges.

My music choice.

No chatter in the theatre.

Skin-to-skin with my baby immediately after birth, breastfeeding if possible

My partner will support the baby on my chest.

Cord clamp delay until it stops pulsing and turns white.

You may label my baby and give (or not give) Vitamin K whilst the baby is on my chest.

Save the placenta into the bag I have labelled.

Delay cleaning and weighing my baby until we are ready after skin-to-skin.

~~~~~~~~~~~~~

Talk to an independent midwife (IM)

Most Independent Midwives offer an initial appointment or birth reflection service for a small fee, where you can talk through your previous experience and help you plan for the next, even if you don't employ them for your pregnancy and birth. (*See www.imuk.org.uk.*)

You might change your mind

It is perfectly OK for you to change your mind at any time – talk to your midwives and doctors, keep a dialogue open with them. Examples of changing your mind might be – changing your place of birth, whether to have pain relief or the type of pain relief, whether to have a caesarean section etc. It's fine – you can change your mind as many times as you like! It is your right.

Your pregnancy

You may need to think about who you have to support you whilst you are pregnant – be up front and ask two or three people to be available for you and try to avoid anyone who is going to be negative or anyone who fusses too much (unless you like being fussed over of course!). You will need people you can turn to and trust. You may find it helpful to be in the company of other pregnant women, or you may want to avoid them.

If you have an overwhelming feeling that you're not like everyone else who is pregnant because you find it difficult to share your 'bad' story but impossible not to acknowledge it, your midwife or the NCT may be able to put you in touch with other people who have been through a similar experience and are willing to support you.

Your pregnancy may well be stressful, so having a list of things or activities you enjoy can help you relax, such as listening to gentle music, walking in nature, cuddling your pet, putting your feet up every afternoon, having a massage or practising yoga or hypnobirthing – whatever it is that calms you.

Towards the end of your pregnancy you might want to 'shrink your world', to turn off the news, avoid annoying people and the phone, and to 'rest and nest' instead. At this time it is possible you will be hurried to start labour, your due date will become overly important and you may feel very stressed. We don't have a word for 'the waiting time', but in Germany they call it *Zwischen*, meaning 'between'. It is a time for you, and your partner, to slow right down, stop worrying and enjoy the last days before your baby appears. Hormones are flowing round your body, all getting into action to do their job – this is a time of waiting and patience – a time of *Zwischen*.

Your birth partner(s)

Think about who the best person or people will be for you and your baby. Will you choose them from the ones who understand what happened to you and support you and who back 'My Birthing Decisions' (*see page 94*); and who will speak for you whilst you are in labour reiterating to the midwives and doctors whatever decisions you have made or make? If you and your birth partner(s) cannot agree, it may be due to a lack of information and dialogue – so involve them in the discussions with the midwives and doctors.

Sources of other help and support

There are trained birth supporters available, and although some do have to charge for their services it may be worth considering having their support. Please note that AIMS is signposting you to a range of birth supporters but will not recommend one route over any other – links to all the groups mentioned below can be found on the internet, as indicated.

Doulas

These are usually women, experienced and trained, who provide continuous support to the whole family throughout pregnancy and birth, and often for a while with your baby at home. They do not provide clinical or medical care – they are there to give practical and emotional support, to listen, to give you confidence without judging. Usually you will employ a doula but there are some voluntary schemes, and some work in Children's centres and occasionally in hospitals. Contact *www.doula.org.uk* for more information.

Antenatal classes

Hospitals run antenatal classes to help you prepare for your pregnancy, birth and parenthood and are usually free to attend. Many profit-making companies run them too. Ask your midwife for a local recommendation.

Hypnobirthing

This is a preparation for birth which you can learn. It involves relaxation and the use of breathing techniques. You practice so that you go into a state of self-hypnosis, which relaxes you ready for your labour. Pain can be a fear response, and people find that learning how to reduce that fear can make birth less painful. There are different ways of learning hypnobirthing – ask your midwife or look for local classes. (Many midwives use this self-help technique.) You will find classes run by various organisations in your local area.

The Daisy Foundation

This non-profit organisation provides a selection of classes and workshops as well as group sessions with an aim to supporting women through pregnancy and birth. Ask your midwife or look for local classes. *www.daisyfoundation.com*

Positive Birth groups

The Positive Birth Movement is a global network of free-to-attend antenatal groups, linked by social media. Your local group may be run by a doula, midwife, childbirth teacher or by a woman passionate about birth. It may be a place to make friends and receive support. Contact the facilitator of the group to find out the specific details about your nearest group. *www.positivebirthmovement.org*

National Childbirth Trust (NCT)

The NCT has trained antenatal teachers who provide refresher courses for parents who are having another baby. These classes provide a chance to reflect on previous birth experiences. Use the NCT website Course Finder to see if there is one near you, *www.nct.org.uk.*

Social networks

As you are probably already aware, there are many websites and Facebook pages and groups and you might find a site which appears to meet your needs, but general advice for any online activity is to be very careful. *Be careful not to post any personal information or photos, keep your privacy settings as high as possible, and beware of befriending people you don't know even if you appear to have something in common.* If you experience something which makes you uncomfortable or worried, turn off! It is best to use charities, well-known and well administered sites, government sites and don't believe everything you read!

Chapter 15

Making peace and moving forward

Beth Whitehead, an AIMS Member and Volunteer, has helped me to understand the enormous amount of effort and courage that it takes to seek resolution. Here is her message to you.

"After a difficult or traumatic experience, it is natural to find it hard to see the joy in life amongst the tangled emotional mess and physical pain. But there are ways that we can peel off the layers, separate the facts from the fiction, to try to reclaim our experience and ultimately our lives.

Remember we are all different, what works for one person may not work for another, some things will be helpful sometimes but not all of the time. It's important to pay attention to how you feel and what you think. You are unique and the expert of you, your body, values and beliefs. Birth is personal and varied, so is birth trauma. The only truth that matters is your own truth. It's important to acknowledge and honour your experience without judgment and never give up on caring for you.

Every time I look at my daughter, I think about the future for her. Every time I get knocked down by a complaint response written by someone sitting in an office who doesn't acknowledge my human rights in childbirth and tells me that what happened didn't matter and not to bother them anymore or to go elsewhere, I climb back up and write another letter then send it to more people to tell them they need more education and to stop defending human rights abuses.

You are not alone. We are here walking with you in this quest for a better world. My vision for the future is a national health service that respects women, our human rights and informed decisions in childbirth by default. 'Continuity of Carer' (see *www.aims.org.uk/journal/index/28/3*) is a must for every woman throughout pregnancy, birth and postnatal recovery. After all, humanity should be at the centre of health and care.

A final message from me are the words that AIMS uses. Although we often feel a certain hopelessness about Maternity Services, we continue to do something good and constructive."

It is better to light a single candle than to curse the darkness.

Final words

Try to find your support network as early on in your pregnancy as possible. Think about the words you might use to describe how you are going to achieve this pregnancy and birth.

Take the initiative
Be fearless
Be self confident
Be resourceful

A last plea

AIMS is only able to provide support and information, and to campaign on different maternity issues because of the voices of women and pregnant people who experience birth in the UK and talk to us. We would really appreciate knowing about your experiences of complaints procedures and experiences from anyone who reads this book. We will use the findings to campaign for better responses from organisations who are tasked to respond to complaints. Email us on *resolution@aims.org.uk*.

We know the system is not perfect, but as a result of several high-profile investigations, all organisations have revised their procedures. AIMS needs to know how well these are working. Your experiences will help to keep the information up-to-date and relevant, and we will post helpful information on the AIMS website at *www.aims.org.uk/general/resolution*.

Also, we would be particularly interested to know if the letters and forms suggested in Chapter 11, 'Making a Formal Complaint' and Chapter 14, 'Planning for subsequent births' have any positive effect.

If you have any comments about the book and its contents or the links available on the AIMS website, please email *resolution@aims.org.uk*.

Thank you.

Resources

Please remember that something that helps one person may not help another. Please let us know what has helped you.

Website help for birth trauma

- Birth Trauma Association *https://birthtraumaassociation.org.uk/*
- Birth Trauma Tree *www.unfoldyourwings.co.uk/the-birth-trauma-tree/*
- Dr Rachel Reed – Midwife Thinking website *https://midwifethinking.com/2017/01/11/childbirth-trauma-care-provider-actions-and-interactions/*
- Make Birth Better *www.makebirthbetter.org/*

Organisations to help with rights and complaints

- Action Against Medical Accidents (AvMA): *www.avma.org.uk*
- Birthrights: *www.birthrights.org.uk*
- Citizens Advice: *www.citizensadvice.org.uk*
- Civil Legal Advice: *www.gov.uk/civil-legal-advice*
- Evidenced based information to empower parents and professionals: *https://evidencebasedbirth.com*
- Family Rights Group: *www.frg.org.uk*
- Healthcare Safety Investigation Branch: *www.hsib.org.uk*
- Human Rights in Childbirth: *www.humanrightsinchildbirth.org*
- Law Society: *http://solicitors.lawsociety.org.uk/*
- The British Institute of Human Rights: *www.bihr.org.uk* (*download Midwifery and Human Rights: A Practitioner's Guide from www.bihr.org.uk/midwiferyhumanrights*)

Other organisations mentioned in the book

- Care Quality Commission: *www.cqc.org.uk*
- Doula UK: *www.doula.org.uk*
- Equality Advisory and Support Service: *www.equalityadvisoryservice.com*
- Equality and Human Rights Commission: *www.equalityhumanrights.com*
- Grandparents Plus: *www.grandparentsplus.org.uk*

- Healthcare Improvement Scotland: *www.healthcareimprovementscotland.org*
- Healthwatch: *www.healthwatch.co.uk*
- Independent Midwives: *www.imuk.org.uk*
- Information Commissioner's Office (ICO): *https://ico.org.uk*
- Law Societies
  England and Wales: *www.lawsociety.org.uk*
  Scotland: *www.lawscot.org.uk*
  Northern Ireland: *www.lawsoc-ni.org*
- NHS Complaints Advocacy Service: *https://nhscomplaintsadvocacy.org*
- NHS England *www.england.nhs.uk*
- NHS Improvement: *https://improvement.nhs.uk*
- National Childbirth Trust (NCT): *www.nct.org.uk*
- National Institute for Health and Care Excellence (NICE): *www.nice.org.uk*
- National Perinatal Epidemiology Unit (NPEU): *www.npeu.ox.ac.uk*
- Northern Ireland Adverse Incident Centre (NIAIC): *www.health-ni.gov.uk*
- Ombudsman: *www.ombudsman.org.uk*
- PANDAS Foundation UK: *www.pandasfoundation.org.uk*
- Patient Safety Wales: *www.patientsafety.wales.nhs.uk*
- POhWER (NHS Complaints Advocacy): *www.pohwer.net*
- Positive Birth Movement: *www.positivebirthmovement.org*
- Professional Standards Authority: *www.professionalstandards.org.uk*
- Royal College of Anaesthetists (RCA): *www.rcoa.ac.uk*
- Royal College of Midwives (RCM): *www.rcm.org.uk*
- Royal College of Obstetricians and Gynaecologists (RCOG) *www.rcog.org.uk*
- seAp Advocacy: *www.seap.org.uk*
- Stonewall: *www.stonewall.org.uk*
- The British Psychological Society: *www.bps.org.uk*
- The British Association for Counselling and Psychotherapy: *www.bacp.co.uk*
- The Daisy Foundation: *www.daisyfoundation.com*
- Think Local Act Personal: *www.thinklocalactpersonal.org.uk*
- Which? Birth Choice: *www.which.co.uk/birth-choice*

Specific experiences

- Action on pre-eclampsia *www.action-on-pre-eclampsia.org.uk/*
- Erbs Palsy Support *www.erbspalsygroup.co.uk/*
- Group B Strep Support *https://gbss.org.uk/*
- Intrahepatic Cholestasis of Pregnancy Support (ICP) *www.icpsupport.org/*
- MASIC, support for women with anal sphincter injuries from birth *www.masic.org.uk/*
- Stillbirth and Neonatal Death Society (Sands)*www.sands.org.uk/*
- Twins Trust – 'Supporting Twins, triplets and more'. *www.twinstrust.org* (previously TAMBA – Twins and Multiple Births Association)

For fathers

- Andy Mayers *www.andrewmayers.info/fathers-mental-health.html*
- Dads Matter *www.dadsmatteruk.org*
- Mark Williams, Fathers Reaching Out *www.reachingoutpmh.co.uk*

When a mother dies

- Cruse Bereavement Care *www.cruse.org.uk*
- NHS Advice *www.nhs.uk/conditions/pregnancy-and-baby/losing-your-partner-or-child-in-pregnancy/*
- Winston's Wish *www.winstonswish.org*

Books

You will find reviews of some of these books and others at *www.aims.org.uk/general/book-reviews*

Be the Change: A Toolkit for the Activist in You by Gina Martin

Birth Crisis by Sheila Kitzinger

Cracked: Why Psychiatry is Doing More Harm Than Good by James Davies

Diastasis Recti: The Whole-Body Solution to Abdominal Weakness and Separation by Katy Bowman

Doing Harm: The Truth About How Bad Medicine and Lazy Science Leave Women Dismissed, Misdiagnosed, and Sick by Maya Dusenbery

How to Heal a Bad Birth: Making sense, making peace and moving on by Melissa J Bruijn and Debby Gould

Invisible Women: Exposing Data Bias in a World Designed for Men by Caroline Criado Perez

Saying Goodbye: A personal story of baby loss and 90 days of support to walk you through grief by Zoë Clark-Coates

The Body Keeps the Score: Mind, Brain and Body in the Transformation of Trauma by Bessel van der Kolk

The Compassionate Mind Approach to Recovering from Trauma using Compassion Focused Therapy by Deborah Lee with Sophie James

The Unspeakable Mind: Stories of Trauma and Healing from the Frontlines of PTSD Science by Shaili Jain

Why Birth Trauma Matters by Emma Svanberg

Why Breastfeeding Grief and Trauma Matter by Amy Brown

Why Human Rights in Childbirth Matter by Rebecca Schiller

Films and Documentaries

The Business of Being Born documentary *www.thebusinessofbeingborn.com*

Mother May I? film due out *www.mothermayithemovie.com*

Freedom for Birth *http://microbirth.com/freedom-for-birth/*

Appendix 1

Making a Complaint in the UK

England

The One Stop Guide for Complaints about Healthcare in England is a helpful document explaining the process of making a complaint – *www.professionalstandards.org.uk/docs/default-source/publications/one-stop-guide-for-complaints/one-stop-guide-for-complaints-about-healthcare-in-england.pdf*. You can also complain to the organisation which 'bought' the service or care you received i.e. your local Commissioning Board or NHS England. You can find a list of the local Commissioning Boards on *www.england.nhs.uk/ccg-details/*. NHS England also commissions some services, but not usually maternity services.

If your issue is not resolved you can refer your complaint to the Parliamentary and Health Service Ombudsman for further investigation at *www.ombudsman.org.uk*.

Getting help with making a complaint

Support is available for you. In the first instance contact your local council or Healthwatch organisation *www.healthwatch.co.uk* and ask for independent NHS complaints advocacy services in your area*.

You can also contact your local Citizens Advice or look up on their website how to complain *www.citizensadvice.org.uk*.

In addition, most hospitals have a Patient Advice and Liaison Service (PALS) who provide confidential advice, support and information to patients, their families and carers. *www.nhs.uk/Service-Search/Patient-advice-and-liaison-services-(PALS)/LocationSearch/363*

*There are several websites of organisations offering help and support to anyone wanting to make a complaint, but they might be particularly helpful for someone who is disabled or has mental health problems:

NHS Complaints Advocacy *http://nhscomplaintsadvocacy.org*

SEAP Advocacy *www.seap.org.uk/services/nhs-complaints-advocacy/*

POhWER *www.pohwer.net/nhs-complaints-advocacy/*

Scotland

You can give feedback about your care to Healthcare Improvement Scotland *www.healthcareimprovementscotland.org*.

The One Stop Guide for Complaints about Healthcare in Scotland gives a good explanation of how to complain and where to look for further information – *www.professionalstandards.org.uk/docs/default-source/publications/one-stop-guide-for-complaints/one-stop-guide-for-complaints-about-healthcare-in-scotland.pdf*.

If your issue is not resolved you can refer your complaint to the Scottish Public Services Ombudsman for further investigation, *www.spso.org.uk/contact-us.*

Getting help with making a complaint

- You can get advice and support from your local Community Health Council.
- The Patient Advice and Support Service (PASS) is delivered by Citizens Advice Scotland. Look up on their website how to complain *www.citizensadvice.org.uk/scotland.*
- Scottish Independent Advocacy Alliance provides independent advocacy for those who find it hard to get their voice heard. *www.siaa.org.uk.*
- Scottish Government website also has useful information, *www.mygov.scot/nhs-complaintsl.*

Wales

You can give feedback and concerns about your care to Healthcare Inspectorate Wales. *http://hiw.org.uk*

The One Stop Guide for Complaints about Healthcare in Wales can be found in *www.professionalstandards.org.uk/docs/default-source/publications/one-stop-guide-for-complaints/one-stop-guide-for-complaints-about-healthcare-in-wales.pdf*

The NHS system for dealing with complaints, claims and incidents (collectively known as concerns) in Wales is called Putting Things Right. *www.nhsdirect.wales.nhs.uk/encyclopaedia/c/article/complaints*

If you have a complaint about the hospital or community services you should write to the Concerns Team in the local Health Board or NHS Trust. If your complaint is about a GP contact your local Health Board. NHS Direct Wales can give you details, *www.nhsdirect.wales.nhs.uk*.

If your issue is not resolved you can refer your complaint to the Health Service Ombudsman Wales for further investigation, *ask@ombudsman-wales.org.uk*.

Getting help with making a complaint

Wales has Community Health Councils which perform a similar task to the Patient Support and Liaison Service in England. Find your local one here, *www.nhsdirect.wales.nhs.uk/localservices/communityhealthcouncils/*. You can get advice and support from your local Community Health Council at *www.communityhealthcouncils.org.uk*.

You can contact Citizens Advice or look up on their website how to complain *www.citizensadvice.org.uk* (same organisation as England).

Northern Ireland

You can raise a concern or complaint about your care to The Regulation and Quality Improvement Authority *www.rqia.org.uk.*

The One Stop Guide for Complaints in Healthcare in Northern Ireland can be found on *www.professionalstandards.org.uk/docs/default-source/publications/ one-stop-guide-for-complaints/one-stop-guide-for-complaints-about-healthcare-in-northern-ireland.pdf*

If your issue is not resolved you can refer your complaint to the Northern Ireland Public Services Ombudsman for further investigation, *http://nipso. org.uk/nipso/.*

Getting help with making a complaint

You can get advice and support from your local Patient and Client Council, *www.patientclientcouncil.hscni.net.*

You can contact Citizens Advice or look up on their website how to complain, *www.citizensadvice.org.uk/nireland.*

Complaints about Independent Healthcare (private or voluntary organisations)

Contact the person or organisation who provides the service. By law they must have a procedure for dealing with patients complaints.

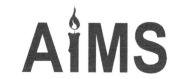

There for your mother

Here for you

Help us to be there for your daughters

www.aims.org.uk

Twitter – @AIMS_online

Facebook – www.facebook.com/AIMSUK

Helpline

helpline@aims.org.uk

0300 365 0663